ALPHA DENTISTRY PRESENTS

LEADERSHIP

CHANGING THE WORLD FROM A DENTAL CHAIR

by ACHIEVER OF THE YEAR LINKEDIN AND TOWN HALL
EY NOMINEE ENTREPRENEUR OF THE YEAR
GRAND HOMAGE LYS DIVERSITY
WORLD'S TOP100 DOCTORS
CREA GLOBAL AWARD

CANADA **Dr. BAK NGUYEN**, DMD

&

CO-AUTHORS

SPAIN **Dr. MAHSA KHAGHANI**, DDS

HUNGARY **Dr. NAGY KATALIN**, DDS; Ph.D; DSc.

GUEST-AUTHORS

USA **Dr. PAUL DOMINIQUE**, DMD, MS

USA **Dr. PAUL OUELLETTE**, DDS, MS, ABO, AFAAID

ALBANIA **Dr. GURIEN DEMIRAQI**, Ph.D. MS, DDS, FIADFE

MALAYSIA **Dr. BENNETE FERNANDES**, BDS, MDS, PhD (*h.c*)

USA **Dr. ARASH HAKHAMIAN**, DDS

BRAZIL **Dr. SANDRA FABIANO**, DDS, MSC

USA **Dr. MARILYN SANDOR**, DDS, MS

TO ALL THE DOCTORS, LEADERS, THINKERS, TEAM
MEMBERS, ENGINEERS, DRIVERS, AND DECISIONS
MAKERS IN THE DENTAL INDUSTRY
by Dr. BAK NGUYEN

ISBN: 978-1-998750-04-7

Published by: Dr. BAK PUBLISHING COMPANY
Dr.BAK 0121

ALPHA DENTISTRY PRESENTS

LEADERSHIP

CHANGING THE WORLD FROM A DENTAL CHAIR

INTRODUCTION
BY Dr. BAK NGUYEN

PART 1
THE DENTAL INDUSTRY

PART 2
THE EDUCATION SYSTEM

DISCLAIMER

ABOUT THE CO-AUTHORS

From Canada, **Dr. BAK NGUYEN,** Nominee Ernst and Young Entrepreneur of the year, Grand Homage Lys DIVERSITY, LinkedIn & TownHall Achiever of the year and TOP 100 Doctors 2021. In 2023, he made the CREA GLOBAL AWARD list. Dr. Bak is a cosmetic dentist, CEO and founder of Mdex & Co. His company is revolutionizing the dental field.

Speaker and motivator, he holds the world record of writing 120 books in 5 years accumulating many world records (to be officialized). Before that, he held the world record of writing 9 books over 12 months, then, 15 books within 15 months to set the bar even higher with the world record of 36 books written within 18 months + 1 week.

By his second author anniversary, he scored his new landmark world record of 48 books within 24 months. And then 72 books in 36 months. By the 4th anniversary, Dr. Bak scored his usual landmark of writing 96 books over 48 months, but he pushed even further, scoring also the landmark world record of 100 books written within 4 years and then, 120 books written in 5 years! His books are covering:

ENTREPRENEURSHIP - LEADERSHIP - QUEST OF IDENTITY - DENTISTRY AND MEDICINE - PARENTING - CHILDREN BOOKS - PHILOSOPHY

In 2003, he founded Mdex, a dental company upon which in 2018, he launched the most ambitious private endeavour to reform the dental industry, Canada-wide. Philosopher, he has close to his heart the quest of happiness of the people surrounding him, patients and colleagues alike. In 2020, he launched an International collaborative initiative named **THE ALPHAS** to share knowledge and for Entrepreneurs and Doctors to thrive through the Greatest Pandemic and Economic depression of our time.

In 2016, he co-found with Tranie Vo, Emotive World Incorporated, a tech research company to use technology to empower happiness and sharing. U.A.X. the ultimate audio experience is the landmark project on which the team is advancing, utilizing the technics of the movie industry and the advancement in ARTIFICIAL INTELLIGENCE to save the book industry and upgrade the continuing education space.

These projects have allowed Dr. Nguyen to attract interest from the international and diplomatic community and he is now the centre of a global discussion on the wellbeing and the future of the health profession. It is in that matter that he shares his thoughts and encourages the health community to share their own stories. Motivational speaker and serial entrepreneur, philosopher and author, in his own words, Dr. Nguyen describes himself as a dentist by circumstances, an entrepreneur by nature and a communicator by passion. He also holds recognitions from the Canadian Parliament and the Canadian Senate.

From SPAIN, **Dr. MAHSA KHAGHANI**, Doctor of Dental Surgery, founder and CEO of BeIDE, a continuous educational platform for dentists. Experienced clinician in orthodontics, periodontal surgery and dental implant surgery, Dr. Khaghani is also leading a team of 30+ dentists in Madrid, Spain. Graduated from UCM (1999), member of the Illustrious College of Dentists of Madrid. Dr. Khaghani thrives on acquiring new knowledge and sharing them. She is the International Program Director at New York University and at PGO in Europe. She is a strong presence in the International Dental community and a leader for women and education. Ambassador in Spain of Digital dentistry society, clean implant foundation and SlowDentistry.

Degree in Dentistry from the UCM (1999), Member 28005521 of the Illustrious College of Dentists of Madrid, Invisalign Specialist, Specialist in Implantology and Periodontology. Diploma in Soft Tissue Management in Implantology taught by Dr. Sascha Jovanovic at the Branemark Center in Lleida (2011). Advanced continuing education in Implantology and Periodontology from New York University (NY 2009-2010). Diploma in advanced periodontics from the UCM (2010). Advanced treatments in periodontics and implantology. (2010), Advanced Course on Surgical Techniques and Aesthetic Implantology, Dr. Markus Hürzeler and Dr. Otto Zuhr. (2009), Esthetic surgery in Periodontal and implant dentistry, Dr. Markus Hürzeler and Dr. Otto Zuhr. (2009), Advanced Implantology course. Dr. Padrós. (2007), Implantology and Tissue Regeneration. Straumann. (2007), Oral Implant surgery course. European Dental Institute. (2006), Aesthetic Implantology and Oral Rehabilitation course. Dr. Julian Cuesta. (2006), Course on Porcelain Veneers and Aesthetic anterior groups. Dr. José A. from Rábago Vega. Ceosa. (2003-2004), Expert in Straight arch Orthodontics, Cervera (2001-2003), Dental Treatment in Special Patients. (2000), Numerous continuing training courses by different lecturers, nationally and internationally. Member of SEPES, SEPA, SE

From HUNGARY, **Dr. & Prof. KATALIN NAGY**, DDS; Ph.D; DSc. Head of Oral Surgery, Faculty of Dentistry University of Szeged, President of the Hungarian Dental Association, Secretary of the Hungarian Dental Professional Advisory Committee, Co-President of the Hungarian Implantology Association, Past president of the Hungarian Fulbright Association, Honorary Consul of Colombia. Professor Nagy did her specialty-degrees (in Oral Surgery, Prosthodontics, and Implantology) at the University of Szeged. She defended her Ph.D. and habilitation at the same place. She was appointed as the first Dean of The Dental Faculty, then she became the Vice President of the University of Szeged. Her main field of research is oral cancer. She defended her theses and received the title of DSc., at the Hungarian Academy of Science.

She speaks fluent English and German and basic Spanish. She gained her international academic experiences in different international Institutions, where she has spent a longer period of time (UK, United States, Germany, Finland). She is organizing the most prestigious Dental Conferences in the last

15 years in Hungary, and also she was the President of the ADEE. Professor Nagy is currently a full Professor and the Head of Oral Surgery at the University of Szeged, the President of the Hungarian Dental Association. She is the Honorary Consul of Colombia in Hungary.

ABOUT THE GUEST-AUTHORS

From the USA, **Dr. & Prof. PAUL DOMINIQUE** is a paediatric dentist, entrepreneur and investor. He's a graduate of the National University of Ireland, where he earned a Bachelor of Science degree in cell biology and molecular genetics. He completed his dental degree at the University of Kentucky and his specialty training in paediatrics at the Eastman Institute for Oral Health, University of Rochester, NY. Dr. Dominique served as an assistant professor in public health at the University of Kentucky, division of oral health science. During his tenure, he headed and improved a novel mobile program that successfully addresses access to care issues for children in Central and Western Kentucky.

Dr. Dominique is also an entrepreneur having acquired and consolidated a small group of practices growing from less than 700K to over 2.4 Million EBITDA in under 24 months. Dr. Dominique has been angel investing for the past decade, investing across a diverse group of platforms such as equity crowdfunding, psychedelic medicine, real estate and teledentistry. He currently serves as a board advisory member to the Teledentists and Revere Partners, the first venture fund dedicated to oral health. He's currently involved in a project that is exploring the use of blockchain technology and NFTs to help improve access to dental care. Dr. Dominique joined the Alphas in 2020 as he contributed to the Teledentistry Summit at the beginning of the COVID crisis. Since Dr. Dominique has contributed to many Alphas summits and books including RELEVANCY and the ALPHA DENTISTRY book franchise (volumes 1 and 4).

From the USA, **Dr. & Prof. PAUL OUELLETTE**, DDS, MS, ABO, AFAAID, WORLD TOP 100 DOCTOR 2020, Former Associate Professor Georgia School of Orthodontics and Jacksonville University. Highly motivated to help my sons become successful in the "Ouellette Family of Dentists" Group Dental Specialty Practice. During the Pandemic, Dr. Ouellette was amongst the co-founders of the ALPHAS. He also advances his research in the field of mobile dentistry and makes the practice of dentistry affordable and accessible to everyone from everywhere. Dr. Ouellette has contributed to many Alphas summits and books including RELEVANCY, MIDAS TOUCH, THE POWER OF DR, AMONGST THE ALPHAS, KISS ORTHODONTICS and the ALPHA DENTISTRY book franchise.

From the USA, **Dr. ARASH HAKHAMIAN**, DDS, is a Doctor of Dental Surgery based in Los Angeles, California. He has been practicing dentistry since 2010 and is a graduate of the University of Southern California with a degree in Doctor of Dental Surgery. Dr. Arash is recognized and respected in his field and is known for teaching dentists advanced clinical procedures, as well as providing life-changing dentistry to his patients locally and internationally. With over a decade of experience in the field, he is the founder and CEO of Dentulu, the world's leading tele-dentistry company which was awarded the Best Tele-dentistry Technology two times at the American Dental Association. As the CEO of Dentulu, Dr. Hakhamian has helped to revolutionize the field of tele-dentistry, developing innovative technologies and services that enable dental professionals to provide care remotely. Dentulu's platform provides patients with access to a wide range of dental services, including virtual consultations, at-home dental exams, and remote monitoring. Dr. Hakhamian is committed to continuing to innovate and drive the field of tele-dentistry forward, ensuring that patients around the world have access to high-quality dental care, regardless of their location or financial resources. In addition to his practice, he was a co-founder of the Global Dental Implant Academy and serves on the board of directors at the International Extraction Academy.

From the USA, **Dr. MARILYN SANDOR**, DDS, MS, is one of Southwest Florida's favourite paediatric dentists. She is highly experienced in her field, having founded her private practice, Naples Paediatric Dentistry in the beautiful community of Naples, Florida in 2001. Dr. Sandor is a successful business owner and an active member of her community. She is committed to educating her young patients on the importance of oral health and enjoys teaching children how to have healthy smiles for a lifetime. Dr. Sandor's paediatric-focused invention, Zooby prophy angles, inspired a full line of creative new products by Young Innovations which have been bringing joy to dental patients around the world for over a decade. She is the founder and CEO of GOODCHECKUP is the first Mobile to Mobile, Patent pending, Teledentistry solution that, gives dentists everywhere the ability to set themselves free from the standard care model and provide patients total convenience by placing access to care at their fingertips.

From Albania, **Dr. & Prof. GURIEN DEMIRAQI**, DDS, MS, PhD, FIADFE is a dental professional who specializes in oral surgery, OMF surgery, oral anesthetics, and implantology. Graduated in dentistry in the Faculty of Dentistry, Tirana University in 2003. From 2003-2006 specialized in Oral surgery and Implantology with DDS, BwKh Berlin (University hospital of Charite) and OMF Surgery, BwKh Amberg (University hospital of Friedrich-Alexander- Universität Erlangen-Nürnberg) Germany, BwzKh Koblenz (University hospital of Johannes Gutenberg University-Mainz) Germany. From 2007, pedagogue and lecturer in oral surgery; OMF surgery; oral anesthetics and implantology in the Dentistry Department, Faculty of Medical Sciences of the Albanian University.

From 2009-2015 chef of OMF surgery cathedra in the Dentistry Department, Faculty of Medical Sciences of the Albanian University. From 2010 Master and later PHD in oral implantology in the Faculty of Dentistry, Tirana University with the theme "Oral and systemic pathologies that affect the osteointegration of implants, a comparative study of several implant systems used in Albania". Speaker in and outside Albania in important events. Author and coauthor of many articles in Albanian and international magazines concerning oral and maxillofacial surgery, orthodontics, endodontics and implantology. Board editor of several scientific magazines. Organizer of courses in grafting, implantology at different levels, accelerated orthodontics and endodontics. Maintains the private practice at the clinic "DemiraqiDental" in Tirana, Albania. General director of the OMF diagnostic center Grafi Dentare Skanner 3D Galeria. Inventor of the "Sticky Tooth" grafting material, Co-inventor of the Baruti-Demiraqi approach, a PAOO enhancement technique with hard and soft tissue grafting protocol. Member of European Association for Osteointegration (EAO), World Dental Federation (FDI), South Europe North Africa Middle East Society of Implantology and Modern Dentistry (SENAME), Balkan Stomatological Society (BASS), Member and Expert of the International Extraction Academy (IEA) and Global Implantology Institute (GII), Awarded Top 100 Doctor in Dentistry in 2020 by the Global Summits Institute (GSI) and later Chair of the Scientific Committee of GSI, currently Regent of the Global Summits Institute (GSI), member of the International Ambassador Committee of the Academy of Oral Surgery (AOS), Member and Albanian President of the International Academy of Implantoprosthesis and Osteoconnection (IAIO), Fellow of the International Academy for Dental-Facial Esthetics (IADFE), Visiting professor at the Universal School of Health in the University of California, Opinion Leader of several dentistry firms etc. Major areas of interest include oral and maxillofacial surgery, implantology, accelerated orthodontics, guided regeneration, endodontic surgery, growth factors, emergency profiles in implantology and so on.

From MALAYSIA, **Dr. & Prof. BENNETE FERNANDES**, BDS, MDS, PhD (h.c.), is a periodontist with 18 years of academic and clinical experience. He completed his graduation (BDS) from KVG Dental College and Hospital, Sullia, Karnataka and obtained a Master degree in Periodontology from JSS Dental College and Hospital, Mysuru, under the agies of the prestigious Rajiv Gandhi University of Health Sciences (RGUHS), Bengaluru, India in 2004. He has done his Fellowship in Implantology from Nobel Biocare and also his Fellowship in LASER dentistry from Genoa University, Italy. He was awarded an honorary PhD. degree in 2021 by the International Internship University (IIU) and another honorary PhD. degree in 2022 by Wisdom University, Nigeria. He is a Fellow of Pierre Fauchard Academy (FPFA) ; Fellow of International College of Continuing Dental Education (FICCDE), Fellow of Academia Internacional De Odontologia Integral (FAIOI), Fellow of The Royal Society of Public Health (FRSPH) from UK, Fellow of The Royal Society of Medicine (RSM)- Odontology Section from UK, Fellow of The Royal Academy of Medicine (RAMI)- Odontology Section from Ireland. He had worked for around 11 years in India before moving to the Faculty of Dentistry, SEGi University, Malaysia since the last 7 years.

From BRAZIL, **Dr. & Prof. SANDRA FABIANO**, DDS, MSC, is a Periodontics and Oral Implantology specialist in private practice in Rio de Janeiro, Brazil. She graduated in Dentistry from Valença Dental School in Rio de Janeiro and completed her specialization in Periodontics at the Brazilian Dental Association (ABO) in Rio de Janeiro. She also completed a continuous education course in Periodontics at the University of Texas Dental Branch in Houston. Her training in Implant Dentistry was provided by Nobel Biocare Brazil at Sendick Clinic in São Paulo. She earned her Master's degree (MSc) in Implantology from São Leopoldo Mandic Faculty in Campinas, São Paulo, Brazil, where she later served as an Assistant Professor in the Master Course in Oral Implantology. Dr. Sandra is currently the Coordinator Professor of specialization in Implant Dentistry at São Leopoldo Mandic Faculty, Campus Rio de Janeiro. She is an active member of the Brazilian Academy of Dentistry and her field of interest is guided bone regeneration, bone substitutes, autologous blood concentrates, and periodontal and peri-implant plastic surgeries. Dr. Sandra is also an active National and International speaker. She loves working at the University and considers it her mission to educate and inspire young female students at the beginning of their careers.

INTRODUCTION

by Dr. BAK NGUYEN

A week ago, I was agonizing, looking at my watch and trying to finish translating **HOW TO WRITE A BOOK IN 30 DAYS** in French before midnight. I finished translating the original version a minute before midnight (excluding the extra chapter that I wrote for the 2nd edition). By 1 AM, I was in bed and the second edition in French was submitted to Apple Books. That was painful.

The next morning, I met with the Alpha *Generals* of **COVIDCONOMICS** and pushed forward on that front too, kickstarting the shooting of its documentary for Amazon Prime Video. By that evening, half of the editing was completed. The test was conclusive and we had a green light to move forward with the documentary.

I drove to Toronto that weekend for family time and to celebrate my latest achievements. I felt tired and off. While I enjoyed very much my time with family, I was burned down and emptied by the last sprint to the finish line while I was running low on adrenaline.

As soon as the dopamine of victory ran out, I faced a huge void! Can you imagine that when Tranie asked me how I felt about achieving my 120th book within 60 months, as hard as it was to believe, I forgot about it? Can you imagine? You don't forget about something that big! But I did. We were Sunday, nearly 4 days after I set that landmark world record and I forgot about it! This is how off I was!

Sure, family time brought its dose of oxytocin, but nothing compares to the adrenaline and testosterone rush that I was used to, as I was piling up and overlapping world records… That took a few days for the dust to settle.

Today is Wednesday, a week after the completion of my race. For the last 2 days, I was sleeping and lost, trying to feel normal again. I must admit that for the last month, even though I was exhausted, I had superpowers fuelled by my momentum and hormones. Now, it's just me. The feeling is quite strange since I am not sure of what I want. I miss feeling my momentum and yet, I was not looking to jump back in the race, not so soon. At the conclusion of the last book, I even raised the question of what would come next. It does not make sense to me to keep submitting myself to such treatment…

Well, last Friday, I received an email from a dear friend, Dr. Masha Khaghani about our book together. I told her to write a list of questions to which I will respond to kickstart the writing of our new book together. Friday, I was very tempted to start answering. But a few hours later, I was driving to Toronto and I left without my laptop.

Since my return, I struggled to find footing and to walk straight without momentum. So I slept. Alphas, Leadership, Changing the World, Dentistry, Personal Awakening, and Rise, all of these themes were floating and crashing one into the other in my head. Those are amongst my most precious flagship concepts and now, they were crashing into one another, creating dents, and sparkle.

Imagine your collection of luxurious cars flooded and banging into one another. That is exactly the feeling. And the crashing happened inside of my head. The noise and the shocks were even louder than my own heartbeat.

I woke up this morning determined to clean up the mess. I sat at my desk, opened my laptop, and put together the cover of **LEADERSHIP**. I was still not sure about the title or the branding, so I simply followed my instincts. All I knew was that the main theme would be leadership in dentistry.

Just to put you in perspective, I am still leading **COVIDCONOMICS** which is aiming to save the world economy! How could I keep my interest in leading dentistry? Well, the presence of my colleagues, Mahsa,

Katalin, and Paul took care of that question. Our friendship and my respect for them erased all of my hesitations.

How do I manage to achieve that much? That is now the question that people keep asking me! Well, I do because I am open to listen and to share. Mahsa and Paul pushed me to write this book. Then, Mahsa introduced me to Professor Katalin Nagy, a very respected name in the world of dentistry. Well, I started a friendship with Dr. Nagy too!

What a chance and great motivation the presence of Dr. Nagy brought to this endeavour. I feel so privileged to share the stage with pioneers and founders of our profession. Katalin, thank you so much for accepting to be part of this endeavour. From one friendship to the next, what Mahsa and Paul started in me, grew to become our next platform to reform dentistry. Before the end of the process, we will be having more and more international leaders and visionaries joining and sharing with us their unique perspectives to elevate our profession into the Information Age and beyond.

Back to the cover, I knew that black would be the colour of this book. We need a sense of elitism and prestige to make this one work. Just like **COVIDCONOMICS**, this one is not just about throwing ideas on the table. It is about finding and anchoring ideas that would change the face of the dental industry and to build on them. Building means rallying, charming, and convincing peers and partners.

That is a huge task to bear. Now you understand my hesitation. If it wasn't because of my Alpha friends, I would have postponed this fight for much later. So, changing the world by being dentists and leading the charge for the greater good were the leading themes. How about **LEADERSHIP** as a title and **CHANGING THE WORLD FROM A DENTAL CHAIR** as a subtitle?

And about **ALPHA DENTISTRY**? How about making it into a brand presenting, just like the **MILLION DOLLAR MINDSET** brand that worked so well for me? I did not overthink that one. I just executed the cover and reacted to it. It was perfect. I spent a few hours adding a golden crowd as a symbol, but then I preferred the simplicity of the black leather and the simple letters on the cover.

ALPHA DENTISTRY presents LEADERSHIP, CHANGING THE WORLD FROM A DENTAL CHAIR was glowing from the deep blackness of the dark leather. Those are not only golden words on a cover, they are literally 3 of my most powerful themes and titles.

ALPHA DENTISTRY is the name of my biggest franchise in dentistry. **LEADERSHIP** is the title of my 3rd book, writing presidential speeches to inspire changes in the World. God knows that we need that kind of inspiration now. And **CHANGING THE WORLD FROM A DENTAL CHAIR** is my title and the title of my 7th book, the one that brought me in front of the Ernst and Young selection committee for the nomination of **ENTREPRENEUR OF THE YEAR**.

Even if I failed to be crowned as **ENTREPRENEUR OF THE YEAR**, the nomination stuck with me and elevated me into the ALPHA and WORLD RECORD that you know today.

From **COVIDCONOMICS**, I retained the mission of saving the world and the idea of acting on ideas and evolution, not teeth. Now, my mission and challenge will be to bring such horizons to an industry measuring daily, fractions of millimetres inside of the mouth. That promises to be an even greater challenge than saving our economy!

So, from **ALPHA MASTERMIND**, I will keep my role as a mentor to empower leaders to rise. I spent most of my writing career writing about Leadership and the Quest of Identity. It is time for me to bring these to my peers, colleagues, and industry. Lately, borrowing from the superhero theme was a great success within the ranks of my Alpha Apprentices. I will keep that recipe of success too!

So in short, it would seem that all of my career as a writer, a philosopher, a leader, and even a mentor leads to this point: to change the world from a dental chair! I will start by stating that I cannot do this one alone. I can only share and empower others to join and to rise. But then, I have the Alphas with me.

With Mahsa's help, we will need to start an apprenticeship program within our ranks too! Joining forces for the last 2 years, I have proven to be an Alpha leader as leaders in the dental and financial field recognized my credibility and are waiting for a chance to collaborate. Between Mahsa, Paul, Katalin, myself, and all of our colleagues joining, we have access to all the leadership of the dental industry. On top of that, Paul and I, have the means to open even the doors of companies outside of our industry for new means and technologies.

This promises to be a great adventure, the smashup of ideas, the assembling of leaders, and a great crusade to be part of. And what are we fighting to save the people from? Mainly our old beliefs and entitlements, but even the entitlement part was taken away after COVID chewed us up and spit us out.

"Resistance to change is now simply stubbornness in the dental field after COVID chewed us up àand spit us out."

Dr. Bak Nguyen

Joined by great leaders and mentors, I am honoured to lead the charge once again to change the world. With Dr. Khaghani, Professor Nagy, Dr. Dominique, and Alphas leaders from all around the world joining, I am confident that we will rally more and more interest and start the movement for the democratization and modernization of this industry.

This is an international Alpha effort. Joining us in this first leadership volume are, from the USA, Professor Paul Ouellette, Dr. Arash Hakhamian, Dr. Marilyn Sandor, from Albania, Professor Gurien Demiraqi, from Malaysia, Professor Bennett Fernandes, and from Brazil, Professor Sandra Fabiano.

This is **LEADERSHIP volume 1, CHANGING THE WORLD FROM A DENTAL CHAIR** presented by ALPHA DENTISTRY. Welcome to the Alphas.

Dr. BAK NGUYEN

PART 1

THE DENTAL INDUSTRY

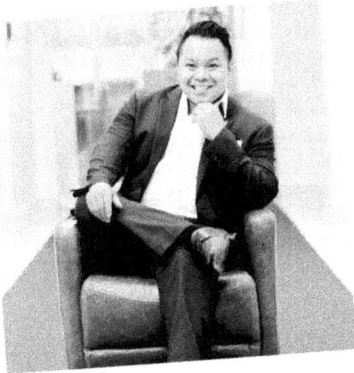

Dr. BAK NGUYEN,
DMD

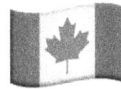

From Canada 🇨🇦, **Dr. BAK NGUYEN**, Nominee Ernst and Young Entrepreneur of the year, Grand Homage Lys DIVERSITY, LinkedIn & TownHall Achiever of the year and TOP 100 Doctors 2021. In 2023, he made the CREA GLOBAL AWARD list. Dr. Bak is a cosmetic dentist, CEO and founder of Mdex & Co. His company is revolutionizing the dental field. Speaker and motivator, he holds the world record of writing 120 books in 5 years accumulating many world records (to be officialized). Before that, he held the world record of writing 9 books over 12 months, then, 15 books within 15 months to set the bar even higher with the world record of 36 books written within 18 months + 1 week. By his second author anniversary, he scored his new landmark world record of 48 books within 24 months. And then 72 books in 36 months. By the 4th anniversary, Dr. Bak scored his usual landmark of writing 96 books over 48 months, but he pushed even further, scoring also the landmark world record of 100 books written within 4 years and then, 120 books written in 5 years! In 2003, he founded Mdex, a dental company upon which in 2018, he launched the most ambitious private endeavour to reform the dental industry, Canada-wide. Philosopher, he has close to his heart the quest of happiness of the people surrounding him, patients and colleagues alike. In 2020, he launched an International collaborative initiative named **THE ALPHAS** to share knowledge and for Entrepreneurs and Doctors to thrive through the Greatest Pandemic and Economic depression of our time.

In 2016, he co-found with Tranie Vo, Emotive World Incorporated, a tech research company to use technology to empower happiness and sharing. U.A.X. the ultimate audio experience is the landmark project on which the team is advancing, utilizing the technics of the movie industry and the advancement in ARTIFICIAL INTELLIGENCE to save the book industry and upgrade the continuing education space. These projects have allowed Dr. Nguyen to attract interest from the international and diplomatic community and he is now the centre of a global discussion on the wellbeing and the future of the health profession. It is in that matter that he shares his thoughts and encourages the health community to share their own stories. Motivational speaker and serial entrepreneur, philosopher and author, in his own words, Dr. Nguyen describes himself as a dentist by circumstances, an entrepreneur by nature and a communicator by passion. He also holds recognitions from the Canadian Parliament and the Canadian Senate.

CHAPTER 1

"NOW, MORE THAN EVER"

WHY IT IS TIME FOR LEADERSHIP IN DENTISTRY

By Dr. BAK NGUYEN

As stated on the back cover of this book, COVID completely destroyed our standing as health professionals, benching all of us, doctors in dental medicine, and white coats, in the worse pandemic crisis of our lifetime. With all the years spent studying, with all the experience and skills operating for decades, we were benched, all around the world to save on limited supplies of masks and gloves.

Suddenly, all of the letters after our names had no value whatsoever. That lasted for 3 months before we could resume our duty. For 3 months, we were left watching the news and wondering about the statistics. But we are doctors, shouldn't we be put to work? In Canada, as in the rest of the world, dentists were benched 2 weeks prior to the general confinement of the population. We wear white coats, titles of doctors, and spend our lives caring for the world! Some members of our profession went out asking for help, sometimes with frustration and anger. They talked to the press.

Well, at a time of general solidarity, on social media, so much hate and negative comments rained down on the articles telling the story of the dentists… It is not personal hate, but yes, there was very little sympathy. It was loud and clear.

During that time, I was in communication with the deputy health minister of Quebec to assist as best as I could. On the other hand, I was trying to bridge the leadership of dentistry of my province with the government, dentistry being of provincial jurisdiction. It pains me to say that we did not show any leadership and we were treated as such by the authorities. And my friends were standing on the government side. That was a huge red flag rising up.

For those of us looking to lend an active hand, we were posted in cleaning duties, because of our sterilization skills… My respects to our peers who swallowed their pride and pitched in for the greater good. But is that really our value? Cleaning duties, really? Personally, I have a whole team in charge of that. I can't recall the last time that I had to clean my operation room myself. And if I need to do so, I will, but I will need guidance from my assistants. And I am sure, my story is pretty similar to many of you. I was useless…

So I picked up the phone and served to the best of my abilities, bridging the communication between the government authorities and my profession. One of the biggest needs by that time was the need for masks and gloves. Actually, that was the demand of the deputy health minister, Dr. Lionel Carmant.

Within one phone call, I had Henry Shein standing ready to pitch in and help with the logistics and yet, the leadership in our ranks stayed very shy. The minister somehow saw the lost cause and moved on to a better solution. I was holding the phone and, even today, we are still friends…

Nothing officially happened, but as the government was trying to face the unprecedented crisis, people with president titles were looking to negotiate… I will restrain myself from emitting anything but facts here. But still, it was so painful to bear. Then, I had my patients to care for, people in long-term treatments who needed follow-up. I was stuck at home and the directives were clear: we could only see emergencies listed by the authorities. The only other legal and official means of communication accepted was the phone! The phone?! Can you believe that? Aren't we living in the same era with smartphones and emails?

I don't blame the leadership in place, they had issues about balancing the service provided to the people and the actual legal structure of our licences. Worldwide, health licences are states based. That is well adapted as the patients have to physically show up in a location. But now, as the confinement was generalized, people still needed care and consults via electronic means of communication, the web… which knows no frontiers… and governments were sending foreigners (students and workers) home. This was a big issue back then.

I could never say that I won that victory, but I have in writing how illegal Teledentistry was by the beginning of February 2020, and then, the same, by the beginning of March 2020. I was desperate. I wrote to peers and colleagues around the world and we came together to know how and how our colleagues were managing their patients. The Alphas were created then as we put together the first International Summit with the theme of Teledentistry.

I hosted the summit through Zoom, from my living room. We were very fortunate to host Dr. Maria Kunstadter, co-founder of one of the biggest networks of Teledentistry in the USA at that time. With us, were doctors from 4 different countries including the USA, France, and Canada.

The Alphas present were, from USA: Dr. Paul Ouellette, orthodontist and recognized as one of the world's TOP 100 doctors, a visionary of the dental field, Dr. Robert BOYD, orthodontist and periodontist. Dr. Boyd was part of the team who led the digitalization of orthodontics in the early 2000 with the advent of invisalign. That is where I met and begun a great friendship with Dr. Paul Dominique, co-author of this book and initiative.

From France, Dr. Philippe Fau is a dentist and mayor of his municipality. Last but not least, from Canada, Dr. Eric Lacoste is a periodontist, community leader and great entrepreneur who is fighting for the weakest links of our society, especially children.

Also with us was Howard Reis, MBA and CEO of the TELEDENTISTS. Well, hours after the summit was aired live, we received, in Canada, the guideline to apply for teledentistry. Hours, after the summit!

I was relieved! For then, 2 months, I was pushing for a means to resume our duty without defying the authorities and without exposing anyone to COVID. I did not fight but that guideline officializing the new norms of practice was a game changer. I cannot claim that one as a victory since I never had to fight, but I will say that I was at the forefront of that one. Well, now that the foreigners are back, 2 years and a half later, we still haven't figured out how to solve the legal issues of our profession. Sure, Teledentistry became a new discipline accepted by both patients and practitioners, but we were nowhere close to a way to make it work. Not then and still, not now!

Everything revolves around the dental chair and the mouth in our field. As soon as we had permission to resume our duty by June 2020, everyone was rushing back to catch up. Basically, 2 years and a half later, we are still operating pretty much as we always had… except for the fact that we needed to balance our ledgers facing the new COVID ever-changing norms, the human resources crisis and the shortage of staff! Where is our leadership?

Prior to COVID, I was working on another one of our issues, our high rate of depression and suicide tendency within the dental ranks. Nothing new here, that's how we are greeting our students in dental school today, how I was greeted more than 25 years ago by the dean and how he was welcomed by his dean, a generation sooner.

At that stage, it is hard to admit anything else than we are broken, as a profession. I am not stating that, the statistics are! I wrote a book on the matter, **PROFESSION HEALTH, THE UNCONVENTIONAL QUEST OF HAPPINESS**, co-authored with Dr. Mirjana Sindolic and Professor Robert Durand.

I even had the federal government to pitch in to co-fund a research on the matter. Unfortunately, we couldn't arrive to an agreement with the researchers who did not agree about making the data public… We were so close!

I went out on my own and pushed for my own solution, **Mdex & Co**, a new way to deploy dentistry to allow doctors to stay independent, to own their practice, but still, to share a wealth of resources that no single doctor could afford by themselves.

The banks and business community embraced my proposal and funded a pilot project in the heart of downtown Montreal. I received the nomination of ENTREPRENEUR OF THE YEAR from Ernst and Young for my work. I got the nomination but ended up losing that race.

For the occasion, I wrote my 7th book explaining my views and how that will change the field: **CHANGING THE WORLD FROM A DENTAL CHAIR**. For years, that was the title I was known for until I became the host of the Alphas and a multiple world records holder as a writer. Today, my company still has the favour of the financial world to reform the dental industry. Is that leadership? I will leave you to answer that question.

"I treat people, not teeth."

Dr. Bak Nguyen

If I will express an opinion, this is my first. In my view, for as long as we are talking about teeth, there is simply no leadership possible. Switch the conversation to people, and now it becomes possible to touch on the subject of leadership.

The question Mahsa asked me to start this conversation was: "what do you understand from leadership in dentistry?" Leadership is about taking a stand and a direction to move forward to. We are talking about leadership when the future is uncertain and when there are risks ahead.

Well, as dentists, we are trained to keep the risk to the minimum, talking about teeth and surgery. And that is great, this is how we keep our patients safe. The difficulty occurs as we are shifting our focus from teeth to people, especially the evolution of people. No risk, no gain. In other words, no risk, no progress.

In my humble opinion, as dentists, we have much depression and suicide problems because we hide behind teeth, taking no risks and assuming that life will be predictable. No blame here, this is how we have been trained. We all know that life is not predictable and dealing with humans, things are always changing.

**"Facing change, one must adapt.
The faster one adapts, the better."**

Dr. Bak Nguyen

And our problem is coming from that statement. We do not adapt. If anything, our first reaction is to deny change, hoping that the storm will pass. Then, if we persist in that view, it becomes stubbornness as we think that things will simply go back to normal. Well, if the change is punctual and brief, you have the chance that your wish will be granted. If the change persists for a long moment, the change becomes permanent and is now a new reality.

That's what happened in COVID as Teledentistry went from being illegal to becoming a new way to treat patients. COVID forced this change. Now that confinement is not an issue anymore, what are we doing, putting back Teledentistry in the closet or bringing it to the next level?

**"No one can oppose progress for long
and still hope to win."**

Dr. Bak Nguyen

I am not sure if that is a fact or an opinion, I will leave you to decide that one. My point is that change is part of life and adapting quickly will make those adapting into the winners of tomorrow. Those resisting behind might be right for a time until they are simply outdated and replaced with better and more flexible alternatives.

Dealing with people is about dealing with change and evolution, evolution both at the personal level and evolution as a society. Looking at evolution through the risk perspective is very limiting and those doing so will miss out on the opportunities built into that same risk.

Please keep in mind that risk and opportunity are 2 faces of the exact same coin. So hiding behind teeth and looking to always avoid risks kills the possibility of leadership in our ranks. Add to that, the competitive nature of our profession and we have a better portrait of who we are and why we came to be so.

To the second part of the question about leadership in dentistry, in my opinion, we are lacking badly both, vision and courage to embrace change. The biggest evolution to our profession within the last generation was the advent of invisalign, democratizing orthodontics. That was a great success story, but the evolution came with so much resistance, and from outsiders of our industry. Today, those outsiders are key players in the field.

Now that COVID shed the light on our place in society, on our public image, now facing a shortage of staff, everything is more expensive, by how much more can we increase the dental fees to balance our ledger? We were already so expensive prior to COVID!

Now that recruiting staff is the number one challenge in 2022 and for the foreseeable future, can we afford to have 3 clinics at every street corner, each competing for the same staff and patient? And by the end of the day, who is paying for our waste and mismanagement of resources? The average of our exploitation cost will be reflected in the cost of care to the population.

In between, we are trying to save the day, again and again, facing impossible odds and never having the right to a mistake, ever! Even if we are the best at what we do, even if we are very strong doing so, how long can we hold before depression hit us? The statistics of our profession are telling us a classic story that we are deaf to, until death swallows us.

For all of these reasons, I say that enough is enough. It is time for us to make a stand and to fix our profession, from the ground up. I am not talking about destroying what is in place, I am talking about embracing change and adapting to it, with game-changer philosophies and means.

We need to do so before we are broken beyond salvation. We need to do before we die. For those of you who think that this is not possible, well, you are right and wrong. We, the dental professionals as we know it, will disappear but the need for dental care won't. In other words, we will get replaced with better, more efficient, and cheaper alternatives.

You still don't believe me? Who would even think that newspapers, magazines, and even TV shows will one day be replaced by people delivering free content on social media? Our younger members don't even have cable TV but they all have Instagram and TikToc accounts.

Even Facebook, the king of social media has to reinvent itself to keep its relevance. Do you really think that the world changes that fast but somehow, we are protected from it? Now, more than ever, we need leadership and vision within our ranks.

This is **LEADERSHIP volume 1, CHANGING THE WORLD FROM A DENTAL CHAIR** presented by ALPHA DENTISTRY. Welcome to the Alphas.

Dr. BAK NGUYEN

CHAPTER 2
"MISSION ACCEPTED"

WE SERVE OUR PATIENTS

By Dr. BAK NGUYEN

With the preliminaries established, let's talk about leadership. But wait a minute, is leadership about talking? Leadership is mostly about doing with a clear vision in mind. The one with the vision is often called the leader and is rallying the crowd behind his or her vision.

But we are not at that point yet. The leader is the spoke person, but before that, we need a clear horizon first, we need a round table of thinkers that will draft the horizon and the ideas before we could start building toward that goal, recruit partners, and an audience.

And this is what this journey is about, about that round table on which Dr. Mahsa Khaghani, Professor Nagy, Dr. Paul Dominique and all the Alphas joining me. Because you are reading these lines, you too, have a seat at the table. It is also my intention to invite more and more Alphas to join the discussion to share their perspectives and expertise.

Without more delay, welcome to the Alphas. The first order of the day is to have a clear mission. What would be the best opening for **LEADERSHIP** in **DENTISTRY**? If we've heard the population, they are screaming how expensive we are! And they are right. If we are listening to our colleagues, they complain about how expensive it is to operate! And they are right too! So, how about bringing down the cost of dentistry as the first initiative of leadership in dentistry?

If you choose to accept this mission, we will tackle it from 2 fronts: bringing down the cost of operating a dental clinic while keeping our standard of living and transferring these savings to our patients. That would be the best formula ever, right?

Unfortunately, this is a simplistic model that would simply involve us going to our suppliers and negotiating bargains. It will take much energy and resources, and soon enough, on the next deal, the price will increase and this will have to be redone again and again. To be realistic, since the savings are not that substantial, very little, if any of the savings, will be transferred down to our patients. More than once, the resources and energy required to negotiate such deals often offset the savings gained by the end of the day. This is too little, too late.

If we are about cutting down our cost of operation, we need to act where the savings are permanent and substantial, as well as it can be sustained over time. I am proposing to cut down on salary, on rent and on marketing! How about that? Let's cut where it matters. But for that, it will require a change in philosophy and in the deployment of our ways of practicing. And yes, I know, changes are scary. At this stage, what is your alternative, to hold on to a sinking ship while the new and big cruise ships are departing?

Cutting on rent, that seems impossible, right? Absolutely not! On the contrary, it is very feasible, if we start thinking of paying rent only on our operating hours, not for the whole 24 hours of the day, nor the 7 days a week nor the 365 days a year! And trust me, that is possible. We will get back to that discussion later on. Just keep in mind that it is possible!

Cutting down on salary, in this time of shortage of staff, is suicidal! Well, the last time that I attended a conference in the USA, administrators were complaining that hygienists are now demanding $90 an hour. That was by June 2022.

I am pretty sure that the next time I will be attending one of these conferences, that $90 bar will be a fact. Even if this does not make any mathematical sense, the market will dictate the price, right? Well, have you forgotten that you are the other half of that market, of that equation?

A free market is about demand and offer. If you lower the offering, the price raises. If you lower demand, the price drops. Do you need a hygienist 40 hours a week? Do we each need 2 hygienists 40 hours a week, just to keep up with the standard of the industry and to provide job stability? Remember whom you serve, your patients. Are you serving them by doing so?

Please keep in mind that from $40-50 an hour to $90, that is as steep as the price of crude that is crippling our world economy in 2022, causing hyperinflation and the menace of the greatest recession of our lifetime. Well, guess what? Oil price goes up and down. Salary never goes down! That should keep you thinking…

And about marketing, how would you like to cut on those? Clinic owners, especially in big cities, all know how much it costs to get a patient at the door. Well, is there any better way to do so? Big clinics are spending an average of $5000 to $7000 a month in marketing costs. They do so because that's the market and how their competition is doing. Well, that too will have to be rethought.

And those are just my point of view. Dr. Khaghani and Dr. Dominique surely have more concerns and ideas to share on the matter of cutting costs, permanently.

Now, how about leveraging new technologies to increase efficiency, customer experience and lowering operational costs, all at once? This is possible if we are willing to rethink our deployment from the ground up! Dr. Dominique has quite a vision on that matter and is surely discussing with external players of the dental field to bridge the gaps.

Who could ever think that going to the grocery, we would be happy to scan each item and bag them ourselves, without pay? Well, post-COVID, that is often our only choice or, if there is still an alternative, the waiting line often makes the convincing very easy.

"No one can stand against progress, period."

Dr. Bak Nguyen

But dental medicine is so much more than grocery, will you say. Sure, but grocery is a priority much higher on the list! So stop thinking that we are better than the world and that, somehow, our licences protect us from change. That is a faulty illusion and half of the population hates us for that reason. It is not just an illusion, it is arrogance!

It is time to open all of the doors, all of the boxes and to redraft our workflow, leveraging today's technologies, needs and habits. But when you say that dental medicine is more complex than grocery, you are right too! Grocery does not have to evolve as much as we do, keeping up with innovation and better ways to improve our standard of care.

And yet, grocery and food distribution have evolved at a much greater pace than we did.

If there was no progress in the food industry, our bill today would have been 2, even 3 times what we are paying. They understood the need for efficiencies, to cut down production costs, and to pass down part of the savings to their customers, us.

In finance, there is a key principle: the more expensive a good, the fewer people will consume. The cheaper the price tag, the more people will be buying repeatedly without thinking twice to slowly become part of their habits. Look in the mirror to verify that statement.

Banks learnt that lesson the hard way, as they collapsed the economy with interest rates above 20%. Then, they went the other way, keeping the interest rates as low as possible to stimulate the economy, in other words, to stimulate borrowing. The volume of borrowing made it into a much more profitable business!

Victoria Secret, the world's best-known brand of women lingerie and Ford Motor were both built with that philosophy in mind. If you sell a high-ticket item, you may have prestige but if you serve the masses, you now have power, even monopolistic-like influence.

"A great means to prosperity is to lower the tag price into habits, in other words, below the resistance point."

Dr. Bak Nguyen

On that, the health industry as a whole has much to learn from the industries we wrongly look down on. That is a great talk, but how? Well, most of the goods and services that we are consuming daily have evolved from the artisan age into the industrial age, led by Henry Ford and spread by the needs of the second world war. Even our education systems are built with that philosophy and requirements.

Then, with the advent of the internet, the world evolved into the Information Age. That again, is changing the field and changing the way that we are producing and consuming. The newspapers are from the Industrial Age. They failed to adapt and got replaced by social media and influencers within less than a generation. That speaks volumes and those are data, not opinions. Actually, by 2022, influencers have more chances to get paid multiples of what a respected journalist might feel lucky to receive. That is also a fact.

Well, in the dental field, our education system got the upgrade into the Industrial Age, cutting the old tradition of having a mentor and an apprentice, and replacing them with university programs. Then, the licensing boards took control to ensure the standard of care amongst their members. These licencing boards are state and provincial-based.

But now, in the midst of the Information Age, these structures and philosophies are heavily challenged to adapt. That was the case with teledentistry and its legality as COVID confined everyone home while the technology was available and cheap. For the rest of our ways of delivering dentistry, it is unfortunate to say that we still have both our feet in the Artisan Philosophy!

I know, you will need more convincing. Let's take a very concrete example to illustrate that fact, one from our own industry: orthodontics. Well, until the 2000s, orthodontics was a field guarded and reserved for the specialists of that field (Artisan Age). Then, Aligntech, the maker of invisalign, came on board and reformed the whole process (Industrial Age). That was the biggest shift and upgrade the dental field experienced since the reform of our education and licencing bureaus. Aligntech got a monopolistic-like reign that lasted for 20 years (from their patents). Now, they faced fierce competition.

Aligntech appeared in the Information Age. But its philosophy and leadership were inspired and rooted in the Industrial Age, Henry Ford's style. Then, another company came and challenged them, Smile Direct Club (SDC). Actually, SDC challenged not only Aligntech but also dentists and the licensing bureaus, with direct-to-customers aligners.

Even if most of us, doctors, will disapprove of that way, SDC showed a great success story and they are just beginning to reform this field. Where are we standing in that story? With Aligntech, we were customers, despite all their branding and public relation campaigns, we are simply customers to Aligntech. Well, the story does not end here. Since the whole revolution happened in the Information Age, the next trend is to have dentists to 3D print their own aligners! That would be the best comeback for dentists, right?

What makes you think that dentists and orthodontists will have the monopoly on that technology? Actually, we are lacking far behind in our knowledge of 3D printing! So in this time and age, tech-savvy people can print their aligners from home, bypassing all of the distribution systems. The more people will do so, the more information will be available and the better and easier it will be to do so. You still don't believe me?

By the end of the 90s, Steve Jobs visited Disney to renegotiate Pixar's partnership with Disney. While walking around the studio with Jeffrey Katzenberg, the studio executive who will, later on, become a co-founder of

Dreamworks Studio, Steve Jobs got the idea of putting the means for everyone in the world to make movies.

That took 10 years and everyone with an iPhone could have the means to film and edit a home movie with ease. That was the first iPhone ever. Now at the dawn of the iPhone 14, some filmmakers are using their iPhones to shoot entire productions. The content on social media is almost exclusively made from smartphones (filmed and edited). That may be amateurish to some studio executives, but it was enough to take down the newspaper giants, the magazine establishment and the TV stations are now fighting for their life.

Well, Steve Jobs did not have any interest in medicine. He died before he could do so. People close to him reported that looking at the instruments keeping him alive in the hospital was painful to him, to see and evaluate how inefficient there were in design, use and etc.

Well, Apple did not revolutionize the medical or dental field, but other players like Aligntech did. And it is just the beginning. They successfully do so because they understood technology and price. They give more means while democratizing the process, both in cost and skills. Their success is based on pricing into habits. And be careful procrastinating, that change happened within 25 years, both the democratization of media and of orthodontics.

"For success, price for habits."

Dr. Bak Nguyen

So within our goals, it would be to bring in new technologies that will democratize (better serve our patients) and, at the same time, decrease the tag prize coming with it or, at least, to not increase the already heavy tag price of our actual fees. To achieve such results, we will need to broaden our views and stop seeing the companies and their innovations as foes at the door. We need to welcome the partnership and develop the future with them and their technologies, shifting the paradigm from customers - suppliers to partners.

You'll be surprised how open the leadership of these companies to welcome us, if we can think at their level, beyond risks and insecurities. Let me put it differently, if there is no risk, there is no innovation, therefore, you are just repackaging the past. Once success is established, if you are not a partner prior to the success, you are a customer. That is the hard lesson that History keeps teaching us and that we failed repeatedly to understand. That is the mission that I am accepting in front of you: to draft ways and plans to decrease our operational expenses and to keep improving of the democratization and the implantation of innovation while keeping the tag price as is or even lowering it. We serve our patients, we must never forget that.

"I treat people and populations, not teeth."

Dr. Bak Nguyen

That would be my updated statement as I am accepting this mission, hosting the Alphas' round table for the discussions ahead, to empower the dialogue and the bridges with existing partners and outsiders of our industries, to push the boundaries to learn from other industries and to include our patients in the process.

It won't be easy and will surely be a wild ride, but with Alphas like Dr. Khaghani, Professor Nagy, and Dr. Dominique to lead the charge, this promises to be very interesting. And with you joining us, this will be more than a discussion but the bridge to our future.

This is **LEADERSHIP volume 1, CHANGING THE WORLD FROM A DENTAL CHAIR** presented by ALPHA DENTISTRY. Welcome to the Alphas.

Dr. BAK NGUYEN

CHAPTER 3
"ROUND TABLE"
CHOOSE YOUR GAME

By Dr. BAK NGUYEN

Now that we have a clear mission, to lower dental costs for both patients and dentists, where do we start? With leadership! The first order of the day will be to cease doing what we do right now since, for the last decades, we are only contributing to increase the cost of dentistry from both sides of the fence.

And that will be our first and biggest challenge. Can we step out of our mould? We are running so fast on our rounded tracks that this is where we will be losing most of our motivation and desire to move forward. Remember what happened to us the last time that the tracks all closed at the same time? We were left bare-handed, us, health officers, experts, and doctors!

In our past history, that is when Kings and Queens got overthrown, thinking that the population will never dare, thinking that a few upset individuals won't throw off tracks the system. Well, think again. The fast and significant adoption of Smile Direct Club's solution is a clear sign that the population is willing to replace us. That is the first warning.

How do you react to hygienists being independent in more and more states around the world? That is surely a growing trend. The people and the governments are looking for cheaper solutions and alternatives. We can either be part of the solution or be replaced while we debate amongst us.

To our orders and licensing boards, protecting the public is their one role. Even if they might not have the solution to lower the cost of dental fees, they will surely not oppose it. To dental companies, just like banks, they know that bigger and better profits are coming along with pricing. They too will understand the mission ahead, especially when about 50% of the population today does not seek dental care. To them, this is an untouched market.

To the population, who would ever oppose the idea of having more affordable care? So who else have we forgotten in this equation? Well, us and our team. We are service providers, very heavy and hungry on human resources. To provide care, we need to be in person, surrounded by a supporting team before and after the actual care. If there is one area that will only explode in cost, it is labour fees.

To blame COVID is an oversight. The only thing COVID did was to emphasize and accelerate a social phenomenon already in place, long before the pandemic: the reserved demographic pyramid. For decades, our leaders and governments warned us about the problem that more people will have to be supported while the active population supporting them is shrinking. That is simply unsustainable at a large scale. We thought that we had more time, but sadly, COVID proved otherwise.

To answer such problems, other industries branched out and brought **GLOBALIZATION** as a solution to balance the equation. That came with much resistance, great performance, and its lot of problems and side effects. Today, post-COVID, leaders and thinkers around the world are reflecting on the improvements to that solution.

But in our dental field, all around the world, we resisted these changes thanks to or because of our licensing bureaus. That did not protect us from the wide shortage of labour, but that spared us from thinking ahead. Why scratch our heads to do better while the rest of the industry is doing business as usual? And we each lowered our heads to dive back into our pods. That's the lack of leadership within our ranks.

To kickstart this endeavour, Dr. Khaghani asked me several questions about leadership and how to launch this initiative. Since Dr. Khaghani is heavily invested in post-educational programs for dentists, her concerns were mostly about the leadership within our ranks. One of her questions was about how should we deploy leadership inside of our clinics and how important it is to lead our team.

Well, I believe that inside a clinic, it is more about management than leadership. Our dental field is very particular, smashing up doctors and post-doctorates with high school graduates serving as supporting teams, with intermediate professionals like hygienists and denturists in between. What is even more complex is that each professional core obeys its own orders and licensing board. Under such circumstances, how can one even think of leadership?

If there is leadership possible on the ground, it would be inside of the members of the same profession (dentists, hygienists, denturists, etc…) but then again, we are scattered all across the land, operating small units, and competing one against the other. It is almost sad and silly when we assert the reality in which we are trapped in. We obey, we perform, and we carry on with excellence. What is left is the direction of the profession and the entire field as a whole, since there is no central leadership.

Governments do not care much about us because we are a small and non-vital part of the system… COVID shed the light on that. So they left it to us to govern ourselves, divided and mounted one against the other, between the different cores (dentists, hygienists, denturists) and amongst members. For as long as we can manage amongst ourselves, the authorities won't interfere. We have been on auto-pilot for too long.

That lack of vision and leadership did not go unnoticed. It became the inefficiencies and the wastes inside of our system. These all contributed to stack up and reflected in the cost of operating and, ultimately the billing to the patient. To justify such high cost, we compare our numbers with our neighbours from other states and other countries and we comfort ourselves by saying that we are in the average...

Since everyone is running the same *zombie race*, the numbers keep climbing and we keep comforting ourselves with the same excuses. Well, the population's patience is growing thin and the most verbal individuals start to burst their opinion of us in the public place, in an era of uttermost solidarity! That speaks volumes!

So how important is leadership? Well, now more than ever, it is of prime importance and a first priority to reclaim the aim from the outdated auto-pilot governing our industry. It has to start with the people we serve and the people we serve with. If we rebuild keeping the patient at the center, we can't go wrong.

Facing the aging of the population and the increasing health needs, we need to plan for what is reasonable from that perspective and to plan our services and offering accordingly. Until lately, we did the exact opposite, pushing more and more techniques and expertise, and simply imposing its cost on the people needing it. That's not just us. Medicine, anywhere that it has not been nationalized, has the same issue.

Nationalization, let's talk about that. In Quebec, Canada, we have a hybrid system, having the government to pay for a fragment of the population (children and low-income households). Well, since we are not a priority, these programs are barely keeping up with the evolution of care and of cost. Nowadays, these programs are often limiting factors to the actual standard of care. So no, nationalization is not a good solution either. It just gives the false illusion of fairness while compromising on care.

I might have shocked many of you, but here is an example. In 2022, if you have a tooth with endodontic need, what do you do? A root canal, a post and a crown is our standard of care, right? Well, under the provincial dental coverage of the province of Quebec in 2022, the extraction of that tooth is the only permitted treatment. Extraction and then, denture (partial or complete). That is simply malpractice, plain and simple! But our lack of leadership and the lack of interest of our governments made it into accepted reality. And we obey!

Just to make it absolutely clear, I am not blaming the governments and their programs. I understand budgeting and priorities. And blaming them, once again, will be a double down on our lack of leadership. What I am saying is that we have to find a better solution.

The quest for justice and equality is surely a noble one, but more often, Greed has proven to be much more resilient and efficient to further a cause. In our Western society, we call Greed the free market and freedom. That's capitalism. I suggest we take the same approach to fix our broken system.

So other than the governments and our licensing boards who are holding the aim of direction, who else have the resources to course-correct our trajectory? Well, our competition! Big tech and well-funded companies have deeper pockets than our governments. They operate based on opportunity and profit, but they understand markets, deployment and management, much better than governments, licensing boards, and surely, our own administrative teams.

They have the resources and the will. The population is screaming for change. And since our license only protects our exclusive right to practice dental medicine from other individuals living in the same state or province, that does not do much in this time and age, as technology has scattered all borders and where technology and Artificial Intelligence are gaining traction, faster and faster.

On Artificial Intelligence, do you know that most governments are now betting on these advances to bridge the lack of manual labour ahead? Keep doing what you do and fighting amongst ourselves and you will have never seen the tsunami hitting, until you are completely submerged.

Unfortunately, I am stating facts, not opinions. Because I am an entrepreneur and that I am also active in other fields like macro-economy and politics, I have such insights to share with you. Every time that my focus is back on dentistry, I have a hard time adjusting, since we are so far behind and we have no idea of the cliff ahead.

I believe that change must come with the patient on and at the centre of the round table. Thinkers, leaders, doctors, white coats, innovators, and entrepreneurs should be at that table to exchange. Each is free to pursue his or her solution, for as long as the needs of the patients are well in focus. As we build on greed and the promise of wealth for the ones with better solutions, solutions will start raining down. Now, we need to test these innovations and the patients will vote, at the end of the day.

I know how scary that may sound to many of you. Well, look at the present condition of our industry and you will see much worse for much less.

Transparency will be the key in this new era. As doctors, we still have the trust of the general population, and therefore, act as ambassadors. As doctors, we understand the operation on the ground and can help the implantation of new technologies and solutions. We can still be vital actors for changes and improvements, in opposition to being the dominating declining class to be replaced.

Not all will agree with my words here. I understand and respect your opinion. I am not progress nor change, just the light bearer on the oversight of our industry and profession. This will happen, on what side of the trade will you stand is up to you.

I will surely hope that some of you, if not many, will be joining the round table to discuss the future and to start bridging the gaps. Our leadership is not about giving orders but about leading by example, of swallowing our pride and individualism, of refusing to keep serving blindly, and joining forces with those with the means to make an impact.

I can't state that enough: change is coming and will not stop for anyone. Our actual system of governance does not have the power to stand that shift of change and progress. Keep in mind that the power behind our actual system of governance is governmental based. Well, the government is betting on technology to bridge their biggest concern (labour) that will fit their budget (lowering cost).

"I treat people, not teeth."

Dr. Bak Nguyen

So doctors, have you chosen your side yet? Where would you stand in the reform of society post-COVID, in permanent staff shortage and in non-stopping increasing wages? Please remember whom you serve and serve them. If you keep that in mind and in heart, it should not be complicated to rally partners and patients around the table and to start exercising your leadership, one in which competing is the small game, one in which winning means to make others win, and one in which being a doctor in dental medicine means to be the care provider for more than teeth.

This is **LEADERSHIP volume 1, CHANGING THE WORLD FROM A DENTAL CHAIR** presented by ALPHA DENTISTRY. Welcome to the Alphas.

Dr. BAK NGUYEN

CHAPTER 4

"EDUCATION"

A SHIFT OF PARADIGM IS NEEDED

By Dr. BAK NGUYEN

In our mission to lead and lower dental costs, what is the role of education? Well, education is the spine of our profession, but I really believe that we need to change our approach. Since we are averse to risk and only praise (and teach) what has been proven times and times over, education cannot play a front role in leadership, at least not in the actual crisis of leadership.

To face our actual crisis, we need to see ahead and embrace the new, which is risky and won't pass any educational standard. We can't teach what we are not sure yet. That said, our universities have much resources and they could be the best players in data gathering, before and after any initiative.

In our field, universities are still the institution with the biggest means for research and could lay ahead the problems based on facts and statistics, allowing the other players of the industry to narrow down the possible causes to address.

Then, the universities could be running reports and researches on the field (financed by the innovative companies) to evaluate the efficiency of the new technologies or philosophies of practice.

It is important to start identifying the strength of each organization. Universities have the brains and manpower, they have the reputation, but they lack the infrastructure to bring products and services to the market. Companies in quest of profit, on the other hand, have that capability and motivation. Once a need is clearly identified, they will invest much more resources into finding a solution. Then, they will have to sell that solution, which will cost even more resources.

If they team up with the universities that brought them the problem in the first place, as a partnership, they can couple their forces to reach more effectively and in a more sustainable way, the deployment of the new solution. As such, the companies are reducing its risks of deployment and gaining from their association with the universities. The universities will be having more and more applied research in the field and will grow their reputation and dividends. They will share a part of the profits of the new commercial success.

I worked in the past with governments and universities, being a company. Well, the actual problem for such associations to gain traction is the lack of business skills and experiences of the people running university programs. An idea is the beginning and solely the beginning. A solution is nothing more than an idea, at most, that is 10% of the equation. The real worth (90%) is in its implementation. That is not my opinion but the general wisdom of everyone in business and management.

This is where universities and researchers fail to reach an agreement with the private sector. As a result, they will prefer to publish an independent paper and then, move on. The private sector will pick up on their ideas and evaluate their merits, only to hire a team of people (often less qualified doctors) to implement that solution.

That story is classic and is leading to much frustration and anger, loss of financial gain on one side, waste of time and resources, and increased risks of deployment on the other side. Basically, a company will pay to a university what it would normally cost to run its own internal research and development team. But usually, ego and delusion will make it otherwise.

Nowadays, each institution needs to redefine itself and reposition its role and means in the new era post-COVID. If I was running a university, that would be my number one solution: to renew and diversify my sources of financing.

As the program is achieving tangible results, both reputation and dividends are pouring in. That should attract more students, quality teaching staff and even more companies with deeper pockets to bring home the next win.

Instead, what do we have? Well, because of a rigid idealism and the lack of business sense, our best minds are flowing through the universities, learning about the past, and then some of our brightest will join the staff of a company... And those geniuses with a solution are burned down as they think that they can take on the market by themselves because they are smart. Well, smart, maybe, but unwise.

That leaves the only alternative for them to go out and seek investors to launch their own enterprises. The biggest success stories in that sense is Google and Facebook, which started on university campus. But the statistics will also tell us how rare these success stories come along. How many great successes are wasted because of pride and inexperience?

Starting this endeavour, Dr. Khaghani asked me about the importance of education and the importance of companies. Well, in my opinion, they each play key roles in our system. Key but fundamentally different roles. In life, that could have been the best association ever, based on being complementary to one another. Instead, comparing, judging and ego drew an edge, labelling the otherwise perfect partnership into opposites.

"Every time that you judge, you are chipping a little piece of your soul."
Dr. Bak Nguyen

It is a little more complex than that, but that is a hard truth to neglect. To embrace ego and idealism, and to pass on progress and the opportunity to make a difference is a hard thing to forget and even harder to forgive. It is such a waste when all of the brains of our profession are going through the same training, the same experience, thinking that school is school and after, life will happen.

It does not have to be that way. We've all been there. Having the chance to discuss with professor Nagy, Fernandes and Fabiano is the beginning of bridging this gap. And then. We will need all of you!

A more realistic approach to our actual crisis would be that the most open-minded and progressive elements of the education system could see this as a pilot project in their quest for new sources of finance. That will be their starting point. In the private sector, as soon as they can see opportunities, they will be listening and willing to try. But who will make the first move?

Well, the Canadian government ran, for years, hybrid programs to finance new research programs solely if they were interests from the private sector. I was on the table as a company looking to extend my hand to the universities. Unfortunately, we weren't ready yet.

Eventually, running thinner and thinner on funds, governments will eventually force the universities to do so while seducing the private sector to pitch in. By then, the terms of the negotiation won't be the same anymore… pride and ego will have cost even more. And as a society, we keep missing out on improvements and opportunities…

Sadly, we can hope that this situation will change soon enough to answer our actual lack of leadership. Independent minds from all horizons, including professors, innovators, and entrepreneurs will have to see beyond the actual trenches and to dialogue. They won't have the resources of the universities, but they have their individual reputation and network.

As Alphas, ideas are travelling fast and much more freely. On the table, discussions happen but no one is ever right nor no one is ever wrong. It is about exchanging ideas and seeing where they lead.

Then, some ideas will find more support amongst peers and there is always someone who knows a private company willing to pitch in. Alphas don't have papers to publish, we have books. This is not a new trench created, it is just a patch until the universities join the new era of collaboration.

In between, many Alphas like Dr. Khaghani are running post-graduate programs, which is the perfect place to present our discussions and progress. Implementation can start there, recruiting more Alphas to start implementing the new means and technologies on the field with the support of the innovative companies and all reporting back to the post-graduate program for recognition, improvement and more.

And why would any practicing doctor be involved in such an initiative? Because we are all looking to make a difference. We are all craving to have a seat at the table, to be heard, to matter, and also, to create more wealth. Since that wealth will be created from the adoption of better means to society, there is no downside here. Leave jealousy behind and let's change the world for the better!

So to summarize, universities do have the means, the manpower, and the expertise to conduct field data gathering to identify needs and trends. They can assemble and package their findings as fundamental research and present them to the industry and look to share their findings with players in other industries too.

In the quest for solutions, which often leads to a new product or service, private companies have the expertise to carry on the development and long-term implementation of new solutions and sustain a profitable business. That said, the riskiest to them is the introduction of their solution to the new market.

Well, if they team up with the universities at that stage to test run their prototype and spread out the progress through the education network, it is a much more efficient way to introduce themselves to the market and to do so with the credibility of the university.

Thus, making sense for a partnership in which the university will report on the performance of the solution and provide feedback from the field for improvement at the same time that they will be spreading the word about the new solution available.

To the company, that is what they would usually pay their marketing team and internal research and development team. Those would be the fair trade between them and the university, in the forms of dividends and grants. More than just the dividends coming from their partnership with the private sector, the universities will be gaining more and more traction in the field of their success, attracting more students to their institution with the hope for such an opportunity, to have access to the private companies and to make a difference in the world! The more students they attract, the more valuable their brand, and so will follow their grants and sponsorships.

It is more than a win-win solution, but one that would require a shift in the paradigm concerning how each party sees the other.

This is **LEADERSHIP volume 1, CHANGING THE WORLD FROM A DENTAL CHAIR** presented by ALPHA DENTISTRY. Welcome to the Alphas.

Dr. BAK NGUYEN

CHAPTER 5
"EMPOWERMENT"
ROUND TABLE

By Dr. BAK NGUYEN

Leadership starts within our ranks. That would also mean that competition has to stop. Leadership is not about being better than the person next door but to lend a hand and to elevate them in the process. The more people we elevate and empower, the greater our leadership.

In a sense, this is where my hope is growing for our kind: until now, we have spent our lives helping and healing thousands of patients. We all have the right mindset to do so. Now, we only need to keep that same mindset of helping without judging, of analyzing without bias, and to apply it with our colleagues and profession.

Forget the titles and the entitlements, see where you can help and what you can learn. Mentors are changing roles to mentorees all the time, depending on the moment and the expertise.

"Forget pride and embrace openness. That is the only way to evolve."

Dr. Bak Nguyen

I am saying this because I saw it in action once! I saw leadership rising from our ranks and changing the field of medicine to start the dawn of a new era. We were so close...

A few years ago, I got solicited to help in the quest for stem cell donors. Stem cells are commonly used in cancer treatment and are often the only means for some forms of cancer. I pitched in my influence, network, and my licence, as a white coat.

Between informing the population and providing local access points for the gathering of the test kits, I reached out to the leadership in Dentistry in Quebec. Back then, Dr. Barry Dolman was the president of the Order of Dentists of Quebec. In the middle of August, as everyone was off for vacation, he wrote back to me from Greece to offer the support of the dentists of the province.

On the other hand, I was negotiating with the authorities, led by Dr. Jean De Serres. The stem cells' cause is a very particular one, one without much resources and one much more complex to handle than to make a blood donation. Well, I set the table for both parties to agree on a protocol that would open the doors for a whole new network and resources for the stem cells' cause.

In our ranks, the Order of Dentists was open to help the financing of the initiative while opening its network for the effort. Unfortunately, internal politics got the best of the negotiations and the initiative did not arrive at any concrete solution. Dr. Jean De Serres is today a very good friend and mentor, and what I will say is that Dr. Barry Dolman and the Order of Dentists of Quebec approached this initiative with generosity, vision, and leadership.

On the matter, I salute Dr. Dolman for his leadership and generosity and I thank Dr. Gaetan Morin, the former Syndic, for his implication. Sadly, Dr. Dolman passed away at the beginning of COVID. It is too bad that jealousy and internal politics got the best of that deal, otherwise, we would have established a new network and trend for the rest of the health community working on stem cells. So yes, given the opportunity, we are capable of game-changing improvements.

In that sense, any one of us can stand up and become a leader for a time. Then, as we achieve our goals, to keep it going, we need other key players to rise and take over, otherwise, we would be stuck at that function or it will fade away as soon as we depart. Neither scenarios are desirable. That is Leadership 101.

Now, how about speeding up the process to make it more effective, faster, and to add some fun to the process? Having multiple leaders at the table from the beginning will burst a discussion. Even people with contrary views will find it interesting to exchange with other smart minds on a problem. Since we are looking for a solution, not a perfect one (which does not exist anyway), all alternatives for improvement should at least be heard.

Because of the dynamic of peers around a round table, there is no vote and nobody has to be right and nobody has to be wrong, keeping the channels of dialogue intact. In other words, the score is not set on ideas, but on results.

"Respect much more than pride will keep the horizon for a possible solution."

Dr. Bak Nguyen

The difference will be made by those who will keep pushing after the discussion, those who will find the resources and the means to execute their solution, who will make the difference. Often, those are also the least verbal.

Well, as a host, my role is to greet everyone, to make them feel welcome. That will also imply that I will listen to them. I will set the table, I will start the discussion with a theme (question), and then I will listen and ask even more questions.

More than once, I saw Alphas around a table discussing passionately about a problem. Usually, there are 2 or 3 very verbal people while others were listening. Well, sometimes, those most verbal are the ones to come back with solutions and means. But very often, the initiative comes from someone else on the table, one very discreet until that point. It is really about implementation much more than to have the initial spark. An idea is just that, an initial spark.

As the founder and host of the Alphas, I was very aware of the dangers of pride and of our bad habit of competing. But then, I also realized that fighting our habits is also the best way to lose interest, time and energy. So I decided to empower those instead.

At the Alphas' round table, I made it crystal clear that I am not a leader, but a host. As a host, I welcome everyone and will give them the floor to express their views. I do have the means to empower anyone and to make them the centre of attention between the different media platforms at my disposal (book authoring, interview, podcasts, etc...). I leverage pride and egos to empower Alphas to emerge.

Because of who I am, almost anyone taking center stage will be recorded and broadcasted. Well, you always have the truth of each person as you give them the spotlight and listen carefully. I am kind, respectful, and I am lending you my platforms. Then, what you say will be yours to bear. I gave to each the attention, allowing them to feel what they project and vibrate. I leveraged their feelings of pride and empowerment.

And then, something magical happens. As the spotlights dim, they now have a choice: do they go back to who they were before or do they get addicted to that hero feeling that they felt on stage? That's the mirror. I leveraged their ambition and quest for a purpose, their thirst to matter. We all have those, ambition, purpose, and the desire to make a difference.

Actually, what I did here was to leverage on our bad habit of competing all the time. Only this time, the competition was between our old self and our hero self, all of it, based on feelings and sensations (emotional intelligence).

And then, magic happens. Doctors became Alphas and leaders, having awakened their desire to make a difference. Because of that passion and release of energy, others will be joining and soon enough, a team will be assembled to explore that venue. There is always someone who knows someone. Very soon, introductions are flying and suddenly, everything is now possible! That's leveraging the power of Alphas!

"I don't care to be right, for as long as one of us is."

Dr. Bak Nguyen

That's the table I set for the Alphas. In other words, we don't care who is right and we do not point that out in the discussion. Actually, we encourage people to voice up and express their unique perspectives. Then, as we take more means to push on the solution through the writing of books, interviews and soon, the making of documentaries, facts and real progress will quickly take over opinions.

Back in the midst of COVID, I remembered the international round tables, from Canada, Dr. Eric Lacoste, Dr. Nash Daniel, Dr. Duc-Minh Lam-Do, from the USA, Dr. Paul Ouellette, Dr. Paul Dominique, Dr. Eric Pulver, Dr. Jeremy Krell, Dr. Maria Kundstadter, Dr. Robert Boyld, from France, Mayor and Dr. Philippe Fau, and from Peru, Dean Julio Reynafarje. Looking for a solution to resume our duty as dentists, we were looking for what to buy to conform. Then, the discussion quickly pivoted to what we should invent to bridge the gaps.

That moment made the Alphas into whom we stand today. At the Alphas table, leadership is to encourage such exchanges and inspire those with ideas to believe in their views, to find confidence and partners to start breaking ground. That is what an Alpha round table is about.

So yes, anyone can become an Alpha, they just need to choose so. Anyone can learn and be a leader, to do so, they will need to feel that way. And no, no one is forever a leader. The best leaders are also the best students.

This should be a great alternative model to our continuous education and post-doctoral programs. In my opinion, we should drop the word EDUCATION from the title, since it implies that information is going from the stage to the crowd. Instead, we should favour a DIALOGUE, to drop the arrogance of perfection and to be less averse to the unknown (risks).

In that sense, my hopes are high on utilizing our continuous education structures to set round tables internationally and to empower more and more Alphas to emerge. I believe that STUDY CIRCLE might be a closer term, but again, we are not studying but building. I will leave to experts as Dr. Khaghani to present her visions on empowering through education.

This is **LEADERSHIP volume 1, CHANGING THE WORLD FROM A DENTAL CHAIR** presented by ALPHA DENTISTRY. Welcome to the Alphas.

Dr. BAK NGUYEN

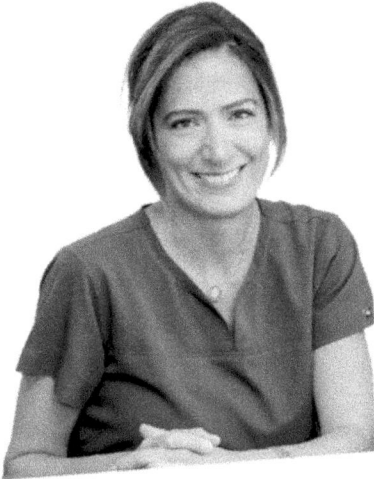

Dr. MAHSA KHAGHANI,
DDS

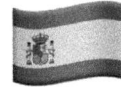

From SPAIN , **Dr. Mahsa Khaghani** is a Doctor of Dental Surgery and the founder and CEO of BeIDE, a continuous educational platform for dentists. She is an experienced clinician in orthodontics, periodontal surgery, and dental implant surgery, and leads a team of 30+ dentists in Madrid, Spain. Dr. Khaghani graduated from UCM in 1999 and is a member of the Illustrious College of Dentists of Madrid. She is an Invisalign Specialist and a specialist in Implantology and Periodontology.Dr. Khaghani has completed various advanced courses and continuing education programs, including a Diploma in Soft Tissue Management in Implantology taught by Dr. Sascha Jovanovic at the Branemark Center in Lleida (2011), advanced continuing education in Implantology and Periodontology from New York University (NY 2009-2010), and a Diploma in advanced periodontics from the UCM (2010).

She has also completed courses on surgical techniques and aesthetic implantology, esthetic surgery in periodontal and implant dentistry, and aesthetic implantology and oral rehabilitation, among others.Dr. Khaghani is a member of SEPES, SEPA, and SE, and is a strong presence in the international dental community. She serves as the International Program Director at New York University and at PGO in Europe. Dr. Khaghani is also the ambassador in Spain of Digital Dentistry Society, Clean Implant Foundation, and SlowDentistry. In 2021, Dr. Khaghani joined the Alphas and co-authored the book ALPHA DENTISTRY vol. 1 - Digital Orthodontics FAQ and ALPHA DENTISTRY vol. 2 - IMPLANTOLOGY FAQ.

CHAPTER 6

"PARADOX"

THERE ARE MORE CHALLENGES ON THE TABLE

By Dr. MAHSA KHAGHANI

It is an honour for me to be able to collaborate once again with Dr. Bak Nguyen, a person who has spent years dedicated to uniting dentists around the world with the sole purpose of spreading and supporting quality dentistry.

We met during the pandemic, when we were all locked down in our homes through a zoom call organized by my colleague Dr. Ken Serota. Even through a computer screen, an ocean apart, I could feel Dr. Bak's concerns for uniting and motivating our colleagues so that the voice of dentists resonates from different parts of the world. I was caught by his words. I really enjoyed listening to him. By then, Dr. Bak talked about relevancy.

It's very difficult to find inspiring people like him, who enjoys every second of his work uniting dentists from different parts of the world to a common ground on which to improve our profession and to find relevancy, to use his own words.

Since then, I had the great pleasure to have several collaborations with Dr. Bak and I am excited to continue collaborating on many other projects together. In this book, I would like to present my vision of empowering dentistry through education. How to change the world being dentists and lead the charge for the greater good were the leading themes.

Leadership to me, is a very important topic that I always wanted to write about. We live in a society where leadership is essential in any activity we want to develop. If you are not capable to be a good leader you won't be able to advance professionally. It's all about a firm stand and a direction to move forward strongly and without fear.

Now, more than ever, we, dentists, need to develop our leadership. In that optic, we need to be very clear about the steps to follow and the objectives to be achieved in order to elevate our art and profession to the highest degree.

To be a good leader in any field requires sacrifices and devotion to what you are doing and to set very defined goals. That is why it is very important to always have absolute control over what you do. This applies to dentistry in the exact same way.

As dentists, we have a very demanding profession. Despite the training we received, we must continuously be in training both in the techniques of the specialty that we are practicing, as well as being up-to-date with all the latest technologies that are appearing on the market.

If we don't keep studying, we won't be able to offer the best quality to our patients, which will make it very difficult to compete in the dental market and to be leaders. Actually, if we are not updating, we are contributing to average down the standard of care of our profession, affecting both the patient's experience and the image of our profession as a whole. Dr. Bak mentioned our public image problem on that matter.

We started with the fundamentals that updating goes hand in hand with quality training. For that purpose, it is important that all dentists dedicate time and a part of their annual income to train with the best experts. That will allow them to offer the quality and new standard of care that their patients deserve. It has become mandatory and required by our licensing boards that each doctor spend a certain number of hours yearly in post-graduation programs, commonly called, continuous education.

This training, in turn, implies that doctors will be able to be up to date with all the latest technology presented by the different world experts. The best training programs are designed to help doctors incorporate the new improvements into their practice.

If a doctor is able to plan and manage the time and investment necessary to train annually with great masters, this doctor will soon obtain results in his practice, increasing his or her number of patients and, ultimately, his or her income.

This all sounds very easy, but it is not. Being able to develop yourself professionally by training with the best and applying the new knowledge and skillset into your practice requires a previous phase, which must be very clear: the access to a great mentor.

When you leave University, you are not clear about what awaits you outside and above all, you are not clear about the path you should follow. Unless you are a legacy and are following in the footsteps of your parents, you will need guidance to find your place in the profession and in your quest to find your field of expertise in which to develop.

Even for legacies, the choices are more defined but still need to be confirmed and perfected. It is very important to know the correct steps to follow because this will mark the future of your professional development.

This is when mentors take all of their importance in the journey of each dentist. Once the students finish their university degree, it is very important, in my opinion, that they can count on the figure of a mentor, who will be the person helping and advising them to know with whom, where, and how to develop the specialty they choose to immerse in.

"Mentorship has to be a must in dentistry."

Dr. Mahsa Khaghani

It's very important to have access to the right master who can help you knock on the right doors and point you in the right direction. Unfortunately, not everyone can afford mentorship right out of school. We each have a particular situation and that is Life, with a capital L. I will advise those dentists to start working and get hands-on experience while saving to be able to access specialized training in time.

In addition, once he or she starts to work as a dentist, as they get involved, that will help clarify the different fields in dentistry and narrow down their interests, the specialty they like the most and in which they would like to evolve in.

In order to become a great professional and to differentiate yourself in the dental market, it is very important to develop professionally and to train in a specialty. You must be able to do this development in this specialty through quality postgraduate programs with great experts, and for this, the advice of a mentor is very important.

Choosing and successfully completing a training program is just the beginning of your journey. Once you are trained as a specialist, it remains very important that you continually update your training because dentistry, like any medical specialty, advances by leaps and bounds.

For this reason, continuous contact with your mentor and your guide is essential so that both the investment and the time you dedicate to updating and training yourself is the right one.

Continuously updating yourself is essential, it comes with your white coat and titles. The evolution in our field is constant and accelerating with the advent of technology. This is not solely for our own personal interest but continuous education has proven to be a must to maintain the ever-evolving standard of care.

Update means not only training with the best, learning all the newest minimally invasive techniques but also knowing the avant-garde technology coming out so that you can then offer them to your patients. You are elevating the standard of care, and the patient's experience through your dedication!
This update through courses requires an investment that, as I mentioned before, must be budgeted and planned for.

It is essential that every year you are clear about how much time and money you are going to invest into training. To ensure the best return on investment, the guidance of a mentor will allow you to select the most appropriate programs for your professional evolution.

With more training, you will be a better professional! That sounds obvious. But is it? You must select and go through the right training programs that will not only teach you the concepts but also help you to apply these notions in your practice within the following weeks.

It's important to choose well. It is better to follow less training and to do them well. Unfortunately, not all programs can attest to be excellent. It is clear that training with a great master is not cheap, but if you apply these concepts quickly, the investment in time and money will give you an even greater return!

To apply the knowledge you have acquired in training, it is important to have the notions acquired but also to be able to acquire the appropriate material and technology to be able to apply them. The big problem is not only the investment in training but also the subsequent investment to acquire the necessary material and technology to be able to make it, a new reality in your practice as soon as possible.

> ## "The cost of all these investments and of all their required material are raising disproportionately compared to our professional fees."
>
> Dr. Mahsa Khaghani

And this is the challenge of leadership I would like to tackle in this book: how can we keep empowering excellence and progress while keeping our care affordable and reasonable, both for the patients and also, for the dentists?

I spent my career practicing with patients and most of my free time both as a mentor and a mentoree, perfecting my science and craft. I saw science and care jumped by leaps into the future. I also saw colleagues left behind and playing catch-up for the years to follow. How can we address and normalize our profession, especially after the reboot of dentistry forced by COVID?

I have many questions to address. I also have many leads to present. With the help of my colleagues, Dr. Bak, Professor Nagy, Dr. Dominique and all the other Alpha doctors ion this book, I am looking to renew my hope for the future of our great profession as a doctor in dentistry, a doctor caring for her patients and raising both the standard of care and the patient's experience! That's my leadership.

My name is Dr. Mahsa Khaghani and I am an Alpha doctor. This is **LEADERSHIP volume 1, CHANGING THE WORLD FROM A DENTAL CHAIR** presented by ALPHA DENTISTRY. Welcome to the Alphas.

Dr. BAK NGUYEN

CHAPTER 7

"PARADIGM SHIFT"

TO KEEP UP WITH ADVANCEMENTS AND STANDARDS

By Dr. MAHSA KHAGHANI

Sure, as Dr. Bak mentioned, our profession faces some of its greatest challenges yet. To have been benched in the greatest health crisis of our lifetime, as doctors and white coats, is surely a wake-up call.

Dr. Bak is looking to fix that, starting with the high fees and honorarium. That is a very noble goal. He also mentioned that for that to happen, we need to bring the cost of dentistry down for both patients and dentists. Dr. Bak, Dr. Paul Dominique and I, all clinique owners, understand the math and the reality of a business ledger.

Since we are acting as a team and since no one has to be right or wrong at the Alpha round table, I will stand up for the dentists. How can we decrease our operational and continuous updating fees?

"The cost of all these investments and of all their required material are raising disproportionately compared to our professional fees."

Dr. Mahsa Khaghani

As I mentioned in my previous chapter, this is one of the greatest challenges any dentist looking to excel is confronted with. While the cost of advancement and technology has exploded, the fees charged by dentists haven't changed much within the last few years.

Take COVID for instance, all the new safety protocols and the new investments required were financed as absorbed by dentists. The money needed for all these updates never got transferred back to the patients. And what about the explosion in wages post-pandemic? Dentists are again stomaching these increases and are not increasing proportionally their fees! If we would, that would be a scandal! Well, we are doctors, but we still have to balance our ledger and budget at the end of the day.

I know that in some countries, dental fees are considered high, but in Europe, and I can personally speak for Spain, the fees for dentistry, over the last 25 years, have not changed due to dental insurance and franchises. On the contrary, they went down. The fees are going down while the operational fees and the cost of advancement keep adding up!

This is a very complex situation in which we, dentists, are finding ourselves. This is an obstacle for dentists to develop professionally and to keep excelling for the good of their patients. It is essential to be able to find a way to give additional value as a specialized dentist who is spending time and resources to always be at the edge of science, practicing new and minimally invasive techniques.

Nowadays, dentists are left to inform their patients about what is available and what is a better way to practice. It has never been more important to know how to convey this to the patient in the consultation and the treatment plan. Then, as the treatment advances, very often, we will need to readdress some of these questions again.

Nobody likes to pay higher fees, this is considering the exact same service or product. Well, this is not the case. Patients have to be aware that the higher fees to a specialized doctor are beneficial to them, their health and the outcome of their treatment. This is so crucial when it comes to less invasive dentistry, more comfortable for the patient. The whole experience is much smoother and often faster. If not well explained, patients will think that it was easy... and then, complain about the higher cost of care! It seems easy because of the extensive training and technology involved.

If that was not carefully explained prior to the treatment, this is often a nightmare in communication post-op. And so, here comes yet another challenge to dentists, having to become masters in communication, just to be able to provide the best of care.

> **"Can we agree that we were trained as surgeons and doctors, not as business people, managers, marketers or press secretaries? And yet, this is the new reality of being a dentist."**
>
> Dr. Mahsa Khaghani

It is very important that you find the proper words and terms to communicate to your patients continuously. You have to inform them of the new advancements in the profession, of your renewed expertise and the advanced procedures proposed as a treatment plan.

You will have to address all of those in consultation, and often, will have to repeat the same explanations in treatment too. It is crucial that patients know and understand in detail the procedures that are going to take place in their mouths.

If you are a dentist who wants to be a leader in your profession and differentiate yourself on the quality of care that you are providing, you will have to be able to transmit that information so it is well understood by your patients. Please don't get me wrong, this is communication, not marketing. You are educating and sharing, not selling.

The added value that you are going to offer your patients will only start when they fully appreciate the care and the difference from the other available alternatives. Of course, by the end of the day, the patient is the one choosing, but surely, most will like to keep their teeth and smile and undergo painless procedures. That is what minimum invasive cares are about.

There are several ways to be able to inform your patients and for this, it is important that you always have the advice of professional people who can help you forge the right message and visibility. Remember, done wrong, it might be perceived as marketing and selling. Done right, it is about informing your patients and giving them more choices and high-quality of care.

Is it going to be through emails, mails or visual information available in your waiting room? It would be for you and your experts to draft a plan and implement it in a way that all the team members will be carrying out the same message.

The message is about the procedures and the advancement in skills and technology, and mostly, about the added benefit to them, to the patients. It is so easy to get lost and to forget that all messages have to keep the patient at the centre, all the time. Of course, part of the information provided will also have to address the cost of that particular treatment.

This part is one of the most important parts. Your patient must understand your care to give it value! And to accept the fees coming with it. In other words, they must understand the cost of their treatment.

Only once communication and trust are well established with your clientele, can you amortize your investments made annually in training, material and technology. As far as I am concerned, this is part of leadership, the leadership that each doctor is embodying to guide their patients.

"Patients will only agree on what they understand. Make sure that they can almost feel and touch the result, before beginning. That's communication."

Dr. Mahsa Khaghani

Now back to the theme of this book: how can we offer updated treatments and the latest technologies while lowering our fees? Unfortunately magic does not exist. How can we face such a paradox and hope to bridge the gap?

In my opinion, dental colleges & associations have to come together and establish a minimum fee which should be respected by both private dentists and dental insurance companies. If this minimum fee in dental treatments is not established and it is not reinforced internationally by all dental colleges, unfortunately, this situation will be very difficult to resolve, averaging down the standard of care and the patient's experience.

Now, the other challenge here is that health (including dental) is provincial and state-based, making it even harder for our profession to come as a whole.

Dentistry is one of the medical specialties that entails a very high material cost and requires constant updating to keep up with the advancement in technology and science. The union between dentists worldwide is important to be able to support, promote, push and sustain an environment where excellence can flourish.

Of course, each country faces their particular challenges and that will be reflected in their decision and pricing. But a dialogue must take place to, at least, keep in perspective the evolution of our profession and industry.

Facing such a paradox, I believe that dental companies also have a very important role and that they could help dentists in the quest for higher and better care, in an affordable and sustainable way. Nowadays, dental companies are viewed by our industry as vendors, looking to sell their products.

Companies have to spend a maximum on marketing and representation just to get to the door. Actually, they are easily spending 100 000 Euros for 2 days in a small booth at dental conventions. And they are present at each convention in every city and country they have business in.

These are expenses that will ultimately be transferred back into the purchase price. It is not only about money, until the sale is done and the money transferred, these companies are carrying on the risks of their inventory and production. How about helping them to help us?

Companies could gain the loyalty of doctors by facilitating access to their technology. By this, I meant that companies are capable of rewarding the fidelity of doctors, giving them easy access to the latest technologies through renting-type agreements which help the constant updating with the newest technologies. By the end of the day, the patients are the customers. Until products and technologies reach them, it was just a great idea… and as time passes, it can become a business liability.

What I am saying is that if we change the relationship we have with our supply companies, we are helping them to reduce their representation and marketing expenses. As we have faster and easier access to improve technology and materials, patients are benefiting (buying). This is a paradigm shift that should help everyone, especially in this era post-COVID.

I really think that this is one of the best ways for doctors to move forward and for private companies to reduce their risk and expense, ensuring better stability for their business. In this way, we can decrease our operational expenses and keep improving with the implantation of the innovation while keeping the fee reasonable.

This is **LEADERSHIP volume 1, CHANGING THE WORLD FROM A DENTAL CHAIR** presented by ALPHA DENTISTRY. Welcome to the Alphas.

Dr. BAK NGUYEN

Dr. GURIEN DEMIRAQI,

Ph.D. MS DDS FIADFE

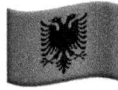

From Albania , **Dr. & Prof. GURIEN DEMIRAQI**, DDS, MS, PhD, FIADFE is a dental professional who specializes in oral surgery, OMF surgery, oral anesthetics, and implantology. Graduated in dentistry in the Faculty of Dentistry, Tirana University in 2003. From 2003-2006 specialized in Oral surgery and Implantology with DDS, BwKh Berlin (University hospital of Charite) and OMF Surgery, BwKh Amberg (University hospital of Friedrich-Alexander- Universität Erlangen-Nürnberg) Germany, BwzKh Koblenz (University hospital of Johannes Gutenberg University-Mainz) Germany. From 2007, pedagogue and lecturer in oral surgery; OMF surgery; oral anesthetics and implantology in the Dentistry Department, Faculty of Medical Sciences of the Albanian University.

From 2009-2015 chef of OMF surgery cathedra in the Dentistry Department, Faculty of Medical Sciences of the Albanian University. From 2010 Master and later PHD in oral implantology in the Faculty of Dentistry, Tirana University with the theme "Oral and systemic pathologies that affect the osteointegration of implants, a comparative study of several implant systems used in Albania". Speaker in and outside Albania in important events. Author and coauthor of many articles in Albanian and international magazines concerning oral and maxillofacial surgery, orthodontics, endodontics and implantology. Board editor of several scientific magazines. Organizer of courses in grafting, implantology at different levels, accelerated orthodontics and endodontics. Maintains the private practice at the clinic "DemiraqiDental" in Tirana, Albania. General director of the OMF diagnostic center Grafi Dentare Skanner 3D Galeria. Inventor of the "Sticky Tooth" grafting material, Co-inventor of the Baruti-Demiraqi approach, a PAOO enhancement technique with hard and soft tissue grafting protocol. Member of European Association for Osteointegration (EAO), World Dental Federation (FDI), South Europe North Africa Middle East Society of Implantology and Modern Dentistry (SENAME), Balkan Stomatological Society (BASS), Member and Expert of the International Extraction Academy (IEA) and Global Implantology Institute (GII), Awarded Top 100 Doctor in Dentistry in 2020 by the Global Summits Institute (GSI) and later Chair of the Scientific Committee of GSI, currently Regent of the Global Summits Institute (GSI), member of the International Ambassador Committee of the Academy of Oral Surgery (AOS), Member and Albanian President of the International Academy of Implantoprosthesis and Osteoconnection (IAIO), Fellow of the International Academy for Dental-Facial Esthetics (IADFE), Visiting professor at the Universal School of Health in the University of California, Opinion Leader of several dentistry firms etc. Major areas of interest include oral and maxillofacial surgery, implantology, accelerated orthodontics, guided regeneration, endodontic surgery, growth factors, emergency profiles in implantology and so on.

CHAPTER 8

"MENTORSHIP"

By Dr. GURIAN DEMIRAQI

I can say that I am lucky. Being a second-generation dentist, my mother taught me everything she knew, starting from my student years. She, herself, had to learn everything, the hard way. 35 years ago, she was the only dentist for an elementary school. She learnt to handle 6-10-year-old on the field (what a nice age!!).

About 10 years later, she was sent to a remote village, where the main prescribed treatments were extractions, about an average of 10 daily, obturations and removable prosthetics. Now imagine doing it for over the years, this is called experience.

When I was a student and saw her work, it looked so easy, but when I had to do it myself, things started to get complicated. I couldn't understand why, I mean, I have seen it done several times and it looks very easy looking at her. Why would she give me such hard cases?

Being patient with me and being there for me, she offered assistance and the needed help to ease these cases. This is how my experience built up. Later on, after graduation, I started my Oral-Maxillo-Facial specialization in a very different setting: the military hospital.

Being the biggest trauma centre in the region with 2 million people, you can imagine what I could see in daily. Fractures and wounds of all kinds from domestic violence and automotive accident traumas, and firearm wounds were my normal.

Most doctors see 1 case of that sort like this in a lifetime of practice. Since the army had the possibility to get implants with ease, thanks to the insurance provided, dental implants and big bone augmentations were common and usual. They became my bread and butter, to borrow from the American saying.

The army has one rule: if you have to buy equipment and material buy only the best, so we used Straumann, Nobel Biocare, and Ankylos implants. That's not all. Surgeons like to place implants but not the prosthetic part. That worked fabulously in my favour since I like that part of the treatment too! Do the math, 10 OMF surgeons place in average 100 implants/day... I took over most of these prosthetic works and my colleagues were so grateful that I did!

I successfully restored and dealt with all of these cases thanks to my training and the mentors I had the chance to meet in my career. I cannot imagine how I would have succeeded otherwise. For all these years, I always had capable colleagues and mentors to guide me. My Master's and Doctorate degree also involved another couple of mentors. Am I done yet? Not even close...

"A doctor is a student till he dies. Once he considers himself not a student anymore, the doctor inside him dies."

Sir William Osler

Medicine is a continuous learning experience and you will never stop learning and researching new ideas and inventions for the sake of humanity.

"Once you stop learning, you start dying."

Albert Einstein

So why is it that out there I see inexperienced doctors performing so badly with things they learn in a weekend course or even worse, in a Facebook big pharma-sponsored group or YouTube video course?

THE DUNNING-KRUGER EFFECT

The Dunning–Kruger effect is a cognitive bias in which people with low ability at a task overestimate their ability. It is related to the cognitive bias of illusory superiority and comes from the inability of people to recognize their lack of ability.

Studies reveal the same phenomenon present everywhere. For instance, a Ph.D. thesis stated the following for those performing complex implant procedures. Those who were 5 years qualified felt the same or more confidence to do complex implantology cases than those who had been qualified for much longer.

Yes, we can argue and debate what this actually means. But overconfidence is a concern. Just to be clear, the current standards state you must:

- Complete a course
- Be mentored
- Have the right equipment

Of these 3 points, the second one is the hardest to achieve. The equipment we use is not a replacement for learning and mastering new skills. In my view, you should learn the approach from someone experienced, before using specialized equipment which may assist your learning curve. Learn to walk before running.

There is no secret weapon or potion, no mysterious formula or no miracle equipment or biomaterial that can make up for your surgical knowledge and experience. Advertising and paid sponsored "teachers" want to give you the illusion that everything can be achieved "with the right instruments", "implants" or "biomaterials".

Wonderful cases seen online or in convention shows by an internationally recognized implantologist succeeding to place implants in cases where it seems impossible are the front show, not the everyday reality. No one has it all easy. For each perfect case, everyone has several that gone bad. If you work a lot, of course, you will have something great to show, but does it make statistics? Can it be generalized in the common mortal work?

This is my point! I know several amazing professionals who achieve amazing results and have great techniques, but when I tried to mimic them, I failed miserably and not for the lack of knowledge or experience, but simply because I was not proficient enough in doing that.

Also, perhaps the case was not meant for that specific technique or simply because we work on "individuals", which are unique cases. There are no general rules that apply perfectly to everyone. Many times, you need to improvise. Don't get me wrong, this doesn't mean, not to prepare adequately before!

There seems to be a rush to provide complex work without wanting to put the hours in. And even then, you will make mistakes. Make no mistake: there are no 2 people alike nor 2 cases that are the same. This is what I have learnt during my carrier, and I continue learning on daily basis.

Please find a good mentor and get guidance on the work you do, otherwise, you may run into problems, even where the problems could have been easily avoided.

"Leadership is the humility to keep learning."
Dr. Gurien Demiraqi

With experience, leadership is also the openness to share back and the willingness to foster the next surgeon into a wise one. If you are a doctor, you are a student! Never forget that!

This is **LEADERSHIP volume 1, CHANGING THE WORLD FROM A DENTAL CHAIR** presented by ALPHA DENTISTRY. Welcome to the Alphas.

Dr. BAK NGUYEN

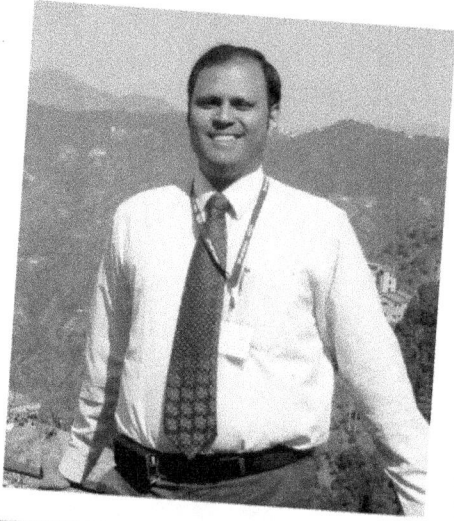

Dr. BENNETE FERNANDES,

BDS, MDS, PhD (*h.c.*)

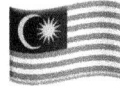

From MALAYSIA, **Dr. & Prof. BENNETE FERNANDES**, BDS, MDS, PhD (h.c.), is a periodontist with 18 years of academic and clinical experience. He completed his graduation (BDS) from KVG Dental College and Hospital, Sullia, Karnataka and obtained a Masters degree in Periodontology from JSS Dental College and Hospital, Mysuru, under the agies of the prestigious Rajiv Gandhi University of Health Sciences (RGUHS), Bengaluru, India in 2004. He has done his Fellowship in Implantology from Nobel Biocare and also his Fellowship in LASER dentistry from Genoa University, Italy. He was awarded an honorary PhD. degree in 2021 by the International Internship University (IIU) and another honorary PhD. degree in 2022 by Wisdom University, Nigeria. He has also been awarded 80+ different awards worldwide. He is a Fellow of Pierre Fauchard Academy (FPFA) ; Fellow of International College of Continuing Dental Education (FICCDE), Fellow of Academia Internacional De Odontologia Integral (FAIOI), Fellow of The Royal Society of Public Health (FRSPH) from UK, Fellow of The Royal Society of Medicine (RSM)- Odontology Section from UK, Fellow of The Royal Academy of Medicine (RAMI)- Odontology Section from Ireland. He had worked for around 11 years in India before moving to the Faculty of Dentistry, SEGi University, Malaysia since the last 7 years.

CHAPTER 9
"MODERN DENTISTRY"
THE HUMANE ASPECTS OF DENTISTRY
By Dr. BENNETE FERNANDES

In the modern age where everything has become so commercialized, where the concept of TIME means money, we have become very mechanical in our dealings with our patients. We do explain things but seldom spend time for meaningful conversations in understanding their concerns, and expectations.

The dental profession is rapidly becoming corporatized. Worldwide, the deterioration of the patient-doctor relationship is the most pernicious problem facing Dentistry. The private dental practice might soon become a thing of the past because most dentists are becoming employees of large corporate hospitals and groups. Some dentists might feel the humanity draining out of the profession — a profession they were drawn to because of a desire to interact with human beings.

More hospitals used to be operated by religious entities, and more physicians were private practitioners. Today, it is generally business people without clinical degrees who manage hospitals, and physicians have become employees of the organizations.

The cause of dental diseases is known, as are realistic methods of prevention. The methods of prevention may change through further research and development (eg, recent changes based on the oral/systemic connection), but based on a thorough understanding of periodontal disease and its sequelae, the cause is known and the cure is clear.

Changes such as these have altered the dentist-patient's core relationship. First, personal responsibility for oral healthcare has transferred to the patient. Secondly, extensive research gives the dentist confidence that his or her treatment is the best possible one for the patient, reducing the old fears of failure due to oral disease, particularly periodontal disease. Thirdly, the dentist has been placed in the role of educator/ motivator, encouraging the patient to practice daily oral hygiene and receive routine professional care.

It is paramount that we remember when we are caring for our patients that they are more than just a task to complete so as to get on to the next one so that we can finish our day. We must understand that we are dealing with their health. What may be routine for us may seem scary or concerning to them. It is essential that we recognize the human side of what we do.

It is our responsibility to take time to develop meaningful relationships with our patients, which will allow us to provide better and more comprehensive care. When we do this, we become an advocate for our patients' dental health.

Here are five essentials to help you become your patients' advocate:

- **SERVICE ORIENTED:** You need to ask yourself whether you are happy with the people you serve, including your dental team members and patients. Think about it for a moment. Would your patients and team members describe you as happy or mechanical? Do you greet others warmly with a smile, especially the Duchenne smile? (The Duchenne smile is an expression that signals true enjoyment. It occurs when the zygomaticus major muscle lifts the corners of your mouth at the same time the orbicularis oculi muscles lift your cheeks and crinkle your eyes at the corners)In simple terms a smile which lights up your eyes. Do you focus on the positives?

- **HUMANE PERSPECTIVE:** asking the right questions to get to know what's important to your patient. How his/her past experience with the dentist has been. Do they have any goals and desires for their dental health. If No, whether they are ready to journey alongside you to reach those. What doubts do they have regarding treatment and what matters to them?

- **EDUCATION IS THE KEY:** This means asking and answering questions so that the patient does not have any assumptions. Also, it is better to have a friendly conversation rather than a presentation. Information should be given in bite-size pieces and data dump should be avoided. One needs to verify the time, sequence, cost, and compliance; in other words, what the patient needs to do to support their treatment.

- **ADDRESSING COMPLICATIONS AT THE EARLIEST:** The discussion should originate from a real place of care, concern and curiosity versus judgment and criticism. Always consider what it might feel like if it happened to you. How would you treat them if they were a family member? Let me clarify, a family member you like (LOL)! Start out by asking, "How may I help you?" Then be present, listen and hear what they are saying. Share with them how you can help them by saying, "I can help you and this is how."

- **Lastly, focus on the WIIFTP (What's in it for the patient).** Show up 100% by being present in the moment. Always contemplate what would make your patient feel more welcome, more comfortable in the moment, and help build a stronger relationship. Keep your patients in the loop by informing them what you are doing and why. It's what we say or don't say that creates the patient's perception. We lose value when we don't let our patients know what we are doing. If we don't say it to the patient it doesn't exist. For example, even when you do a detailed periodontal examination explain to your patient what you are doing and the reasons why. Even for those patients you have seen for many years, even them you need to inform at every visit. The why must always be a value statement highlighting the benefit for the patient, especially their systemic health and not the practice or the team.

To summarize, we must never, even for a moment, disregard that we are at first human beings caring for the health of other human beings. It is not just about fixing their teeth. There are humans attached to those teeth which we treat! It is important that we focus on the human side of dentistry and become advocates for our patients' health by optimizing their oral health.

As an experienced practitioner, these came with experience. As a teacher, I am looking for ways to transfer that experience to my students, because without human touch, dentistry is cold and can be very scary. I did not become a dentist to scare people away. And I am sure, neither did you!

This is **LEADERSHIP volume 1, CHANGING THE WORLD FROM A DENTAL CHAIR** presented by ALPHA DENTISTRY. Welcome to the Alphas.

Dr. BAK NGUYEN

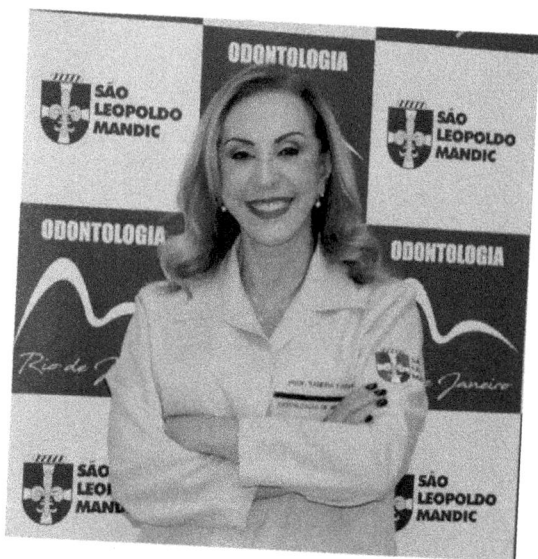

Dr. SANDRA FABIANO,
DDS, MSC

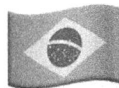

From BRAZIL, **Dr. & Prof. SANDRA FABIANO**, DDS, MSC, is a Periodontics and Oral Implantology specialist in private practice in Rio de Janeiro, Brazil. She graduated in Dentistry from Valença Dental School in Rio de Janeiro and completed her specialization in Periodontics at the Brazilian Dental Association (ABO) in Rio de Janeiro. She also completed a continuous education course in Periodontics at the University of Texas Dental Branch in Houston.

Her training in Implant Dentistry was provided by Nobel Biocare Brazil at Sendick Clinic in São Paulo. She earned her Master's degree (MSc) in Implantology from São Leopoldo Mandic Faculty in Campinas, São Paulo, Brazil, where she later served as an Assistant Professor in the Master Course in Oral Implantology. Dr. Sandra is currently the Coordinator Professor of specialization in Implant Dentistry at São Leopoldo Mandic Faculty, Campus Rio de Janeiro. She is an active member of the Brazilian Academy of Dentistry and her field of interest is guided bone regeneration, bone substitutes, autologous blood concentrates, and periodontal and peri-implant plastic surgeries. Dr. Sandra is also an active National and International speaker. She loves working at the University and considers it her mission to educate and inspire young female students at the beginning of their careers.

CHAPTER 10

"LEADERSHIP FROM LEARNING AND SHARING"

PASSION, COMMITMENT AND A LITTLE BIT OF LUCK

By Dr. SANDRA FABIANO

My story with Dr. Bak and with the ALPHAS started a little while ago when I was invited to participate as a co-author of the book **ALPHA DENTISTRY vol. 2 - IMPLANTOLOGY FAQ**. We didn't know each other, either virtually or in person. We were introduced by a mutual friend Dr. Preetinder Singh.

Since then I've had the opportunity to exchange ideas with Dr. Bak and see how visionary, motivating, and enterprising he is. I am very grateful to him for his friendship and for sharing new ideas on how to practice in more human ways.

The fact that we are here exchanging ideas shows how COVID-19 pandemic changed drastically the world. Socioeconomic problems spiked, affecting both dentists and patients. If we don't adapt to the new reality, we will be run over.

What does this have to do with Leadership? If we think about it, we, as opinion makers, are a mirror for younger people who are arriving in the world, fighting to find a place to stand. Mainly, the recent graduates who leave dental school are totally lost, without knowing if it was really worth it to specialize!

Dental schools prepare dentists to exercise their technical skills but do not prepare them to run their own business nor to deal with patients on a human level. For most graduates, they get are positions in franchises where they are neither valued nor fairly compensated. This is the reality that I see in Brazil, and I believe that some of you will find in your respective countries.

I don't teach at the undergraduate level, but if I could suggest something to the dental deans, I would advise them to prepare, as soon as possible, the future cohorts of dentists to face the *real world* after graduation. That means dealing with people, not only teeth.

In my classes, I teach students ranging from 25 to 60 years old, who want to specialize in Implant Dentistry. In my current class, the students are very young, practically recent graduates. Teaching them, I realized that I am a mirror for them in terms of where they want to go. It is my duty to show leadership and to be a role model, dental-wise. Actually, I made it my life mission.

Amongst these students, the majority are women. Currently in Brazil, 70% of dentists are women. This increase in the female gender is impressive! To understand the present and the future, we have to study the past. Most women in my childhood, despite being exceptional individuals, did not have the opportunity to occupy leadership positions. Nowadays, women have had to overcome countless challenges, just to prove that they are capable of performing as well as their male counterparts.

Today, women have obtained the qualification and recognition to perform in positions that, not too long ago, were reserved only for men. The evolution has been a gradual one, and I commend the women of my past for prepping the way and for inspiring me to walk my own path. Without them, I won't be who I am today!

As a woman and a teacher, I know that I am able to inspire my students, male and female. What I have to say is that it goes both ways. They inspire me too! I push them to embrace new ideas and take every opportunity to grow.

**"Success is a matter of choice.
Success is the fruit of recognizing a job well done."**
Dr. Sandra Fabiano

Our specialization course in Implant Dentistry at the Faculty of Dentistry São Leopoldo Mandic, Rio de Janeiro, lasts 28 months. It is a course in Implant Dentistry with an emphasis on peri-implant plastic surgery.

I always tell my students that there is no point in skipping steps. There is a learning curve and little by little, they will master the techniques. The current course is merely the beginning of mastering a new science. They should continue learning and improving their craft by attending other immersion courses in advanced techniques. The advancements in science introduce, almost daily, new procedures, new tools, and new protocols to make the procedures less invasive and more efficient.

The big upside of being part of a University is the ability to have access nearly to all the newest instruments, equipment, and technology, often at a discount and before they are made available to the general public (dentists). On that, Universities are prime clients to the dental companies operating in that space, because we are a great marketing network through our students.

"With much effort, love for what we do, and some sacrifice, it is possible to achieve our goals and dreams."

Dr. Sandra Fabiano

Back when I was in high school, I thought of majoring in architecture. I believed that the free and beautiful forms used by architects were a challenge to be faced. Then, my passion for biology got the best of me and my encounter with dentistry has been inspiring and enjoyable to this day.

When I graduated from dental school, I didn't have any doubts about what specialty I would enrol in. I loved both periodontics and surgery. I finally decided to be a specialist in periodontics. I completed my course at the Brazilian Association of Dentistry (ABO). For my specialty, I had to show much dedication. It was two years of continuous and arduous study and practice.

Through that curriculum, I had the idea of creating a Department of Oral Prevention and I got the support of my professors and the President of the ABO. The objective was to train community agents on the fundamentals of preventive dentistry to teach in schools and communities. How to take care of oral health was my goal. I stayed ahead of this work for a few years. It was so rewarding to share life-changing information and experience with people who did not have access to private treatment.

"Choices, encounters, and a bit of luck."

Dr. Sandra Fabiano

Pioneer women who passionately exercise their profession are inspirations to me. Learning from them, I learnt to stay motivated and to never give up on my goals and ideals. Dr. Katalin Nagy is one of these inspiring women, her trajectory and life story are so inspirational to so many women.

I got married and as a new specialist in periodontics, I had the opportunity to go to the University of Texas in Houston for a continuous education course in periodontics. It was my first contact with dental implants. Again, I emphasize that our lives are a sum of our choices, encounters, and a bit of luck. Life just works out!

A new chapter of my life was beginning to take place to bridge my knowledge of periodontics with implant dentistry. Back in Brazil, I attended an implant training course in São Paulo at Nobel Biocare Brazil. On this occasion, my desire to teach, share, and get more knowledge in dentistry led me to pursue a Master's in Implant Dentistry at São Leopoldo Mandic Faculty, In Campinas, São Paulo.

With a new Master's Degree in Implantology, I was invited by the dean of the University to join the Masters's Teaching Team as an Assistant Professor. Shortly after, I was offered the position of Coordinating Professor of Specialization in Implant Dentistry in Rio de Janeiro, where the university maintains an advanced campus for postgraduate courses in several areas of dentistry.

"I treat people, not teeth."

Dr. Bak Nguyen

Borrowing from Dr. Bak, I treat people, not teeth! I like to practice periodontics and implantology in my private clinic, but I also love teaching at the University. A teacher does more than teach new techniques, a teacher educates and teaches how to practice the profession with ethics and passion.

And I know a good teacher inspires those she teaches. As a mentor to my students, I teach them that each patient is a unique individual, with unique experiences, sociocultural, and psychological baggage.

"Never give up!"

Dr. Sandra Fabiano

I am a woman in the dental profession and currently hold the position of Coordinating Professor of Specialization in Implant Dentistry at a well-known university. I can say that many times the path has been challenging but as I said previously, women who passionately exercise their profession are my inspiration, and that has motivated me to never give up on my goal and ideals.

My many years of studies, clinical observation, and hard work all contributed to what I teach today. I feel blessed that each day offers me opportunities to learn more and connect with like-minded people.

I'm passionate about sharing my findings with my students, colleagues, and peers. My leadership style is to keep learning and to keep sharing. Yes, we can change the world from a dental chair!

This is **LEADERSHIP volume 1, CHANGING THE WORLD FROM A DENTAL CHAIR** presented by ALPHA DENTISTRY. Welcome to the Alphas.

Dr. BAK NGUYEN

PART 2

THE EDUCATION SYSTEM

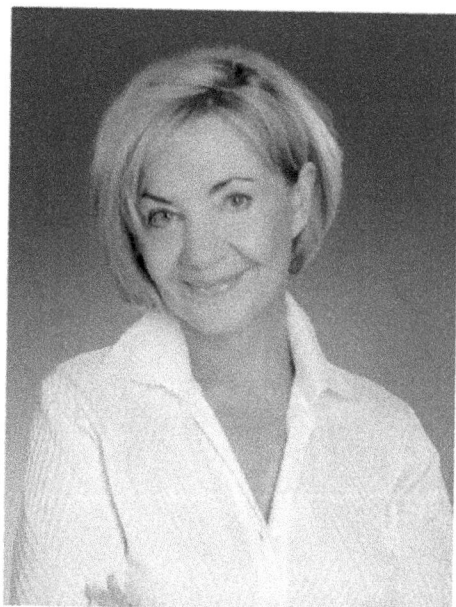

Dr. KATALIN NAGY,
DDS; Ph.D; DSc.

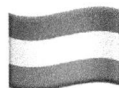

From HUNGARY 🇭🇺, **Dr. & Prof. KATALIN NAGY**, DDS; Ph.D; DSc. Head of Oral Surgery, Faculty of Dentistry University of Szeged, President of the Hungarian Dental Association, Secretary of the Hungarian Dental Professional Advisory Committee, Co-President of the Hungarian Implantology Association, Past president of the Hungarian Fulbright Association, Honorary Consul of Colombia. Professor Nagy did her specialty-degrees (in Oral Surgery, Prosthodontics, and Implantology) at the University of Szeged. She defended her Ph.D. and habilitation at the same place. She was appointed as the first Dean of The Dental Faculty, then she became the Vice President of the University of Szeged. Her main field of research is oral cancer. She defended her theses and received the title of DSc., at the Hungarian Academy of Science.

She speaks fluent English and German and basic Spanish. She gained her international academic experiences in different international Institutions, where she has spent a longer period of time (UK, United States, Germany, Finland). She is organizing the most prestigious Dental Conferences in the last 15 years in Hungary, and also she was the President of the ADEE. Professor Nagy is currently a full Professor and the Head of Oral Surgery at the University of Szeged, the President of the Hungarian Dental Association. She is the Honorary Consul of Colombia in Hungary.

CHAPTER 11
"Dr. KATALIN NAGY"
THE BIGGER PICTURE

By Dr. BAK NGUYEN

The leadership of the ALPHAS is about greeting other Alphas to the table. I am grateful that Dr. Mahsa Khaghani extended the invitation of this book to 2 times former Dean and serving President of the Dentist Association of Hungary, Dr. Katalin Nagy. Actually, Dr. Nagy was more than a dean, she founded the dental faculty!

Dr. Nagy is a Hungarian dentist and the head of the Department of Oral Surgery at the University of Saget, a top-ranking university in Hungary. She has received extensive training in dentistry, including specialist degrees, a PhD in rehabilitation, and graduated from the Faculty of Dentistry of the University of Szeged in 1982.

Dr. Nagy has made a significant impact in the field of dentistry, serving as the founder and first Dean of the Faculty of Dentistry of the University of Szeged and contributing to research in areas such as prosthetic rehabilitation and smoking cessation. She has also been honoured with numerous awards, including the Lifetime Achievement Award in Public Service and Professional Excellence and the Pro Urbe Award for promoting international relations.

She has more than 40 years in academia, teaching dentistry. She saw the evolution of dentistry within the last 4 decades. Lately, we had a discussion on the matter of the mirror COVID reflected on our profession. On that, you know where I stand. Discussing with Katalin, she shared even deeper views and perspectives of how in need of updates, upgrades even, the dental education system required.

On that, we all agreed on the need of improvement to upgrade dentistry into the Information Age while finding ways to make it more affordable, even from the education standpoint.

In addition to her work in dentistry, Dr. Nagy is also the honorary consul of Colombia and works to connect the two countries in the education field. She has also organized a dental conference for the last 16 years, with the exception of the past two years due to the COVID-19 pandemic. She continues to be a dedicated and highly regarded professional in the field of dentistry.

It is my honour and privilege to introduce Dr. Katalin Nagy as she will be leading the reflection on the future of our Dental education system (University) and bridging the dental faculties throughout the world into the Information Age and the Collaborative Age, one more focused on the person in our dental chair.

Please join me to welcome to the Alphas, Dr. Katalin Nagy.

This is **LEADERSHIP volume 1, CHANGING THE WORLD FROM A DENTAL CHAIR** presented by ALPHA DENTISTRY. Welcome to the Alphas.

Dr. BAK NGUYEN

CHAPTER 12
"FEMALE LEADERSHIP"
THE SILENT FIGHT

Interview of Dr. KATALIN NAGY

Written by Dr. BAK NGUYEN

I believe the past two years have been a total catastrophe in many aspects, not just for my conferences but for many things in general. I hope that this kind of widespread shutdown never happens again. Regardless of any future viruses or illnesses that may arise, I hope that we will always find a way to carry on without having to completely shut down. That forced "pause" allowed me to reflect on many aspects and facts of our profession. Let's address the statistics and their disconnections.

Dentistry and education are worlds of men, despite that more and more women are shaping the profession. In Hungary, 57% of dentists are women (Hungarian Central Statistical Office 2016). In Europe, 60% of dentists are women (Dental Economics), going up as high as 75% in Finland. That is why I think it is important to address this topic of woman's leadership.

"The worst thing to do is to make a woman into a man."
Dr. Katalin Nagy

As we represent the majority of the profession, I really believe that women have a say in the evolution of dentistry. To better understand where I am coming from, allow me to share with you my personal journey as a dentist, a professor, a dean, a mother, but above all, a woman in dentistry.

"Excelling in multiple aspects of life is difficult to achieve while staying balanced."
Dr. Katalin Nagy

When I started my career, I had to make sacrifices, particularly in my personal life. I had a young son and I wanted to be a good mother to him, but at the same time, I wanted to pursue my career. I lost my husband when my son was 6, so I knew that the journey ahead would not be easy.

I was determined to be both parents to my son while advancing my career in academia. I can say that I faced challenging times while trying to balance my career and being a good single mother to my son. I found a way to combine both: I took my son with me everywhere I went and found people to take care of him while I was working. This meant that I didn't have much of a personal life, but rather a life that was a combination of caring for my son and building my career.

I went to Germany to teach and then to London for my Ph.D. at the Eastman Dental Institute. Everywhere, my son followed me, shadowed me. Actually, he learnt to adapt from a very young age. Switching environment was hard, switching languages was a much harder challenge for him, going from Hungarian to German to English within a short amount of time. Despite the difficulties, I don't regret my choices because I was able to provide my son with a fantastic upbringing and built my career at the same time.

My time at the Eastman Dental Institute was a fantastic experience and I was able to maintain a balance between my personal and professional life despite the challenges that come with raising a child as a single mother. I eventually received a Fulbright Fellowship to study at Sloan Kettering Cancer Center in New York and moved there with my son.

Although it was a hard life for both of us, I believe that I managed to find a balance. My son enjoyed his time in the United States. However, I do think that a mother sacrifices something if she chooses to pursue her career while also taking care of her child. It's not easy, but it's definitely manageable. And that is the reality that our profession is discounting. We are dedicated surgeons, improving our skills and craft, implementing new technologies, but too often, we are forgetting the individuals and their identity at the core of our profession.

We won't change our profession in a day. But with sensitivity and diplomacy, I believe that it is possible to influence its evolution, and therefore, the future of our profession to adapt to the reality of its workforce.

Having dedicated my professional life to dentistry, here are my advice to the women in our ranks. First of all, the change has to come from within. We are women, we are built differently, and have our roles as women to bear. Don't get me wrong, I am not complaining, just recognizing our reality. We are women and we should act as such.

Even if there is an unfortunate event in your life like losing a husband, I would advise everyone, including my younger self, to marry again and have a support system. This was one of my biggest mistakes. I did not remarry because I thought it wouldn't be good for my kid, that I cannot never replace his father, but that was my mistake and I would probably change that if I could go back in time. However, with a supportive family, it is doable to have a career and a family. You support your husband when he has a career path, and vice versa.

"It is hard to be both the woman and the man, even harder to keep excelling."

Dr. Katalin Nagy

I would not advise anyone to not have a career and just look after their kids. Nowadays, the new generation is much more evolved in that matter and able to handle things with more ease. I am not saying that it is easier, just that society has evolved and it is possible and normal to be a woman in all its senses while being a strong contributing member of society.

With the help of technology, kids are able to fit into society with ease, giving mothers a chance to build their careers, especially if they have a supportive family. Back in my time, my kid did not have an iPad to help him cope. Today, that is like a universal passport in many situations. I am repeating myself: women should all have their support system to, in turn, be the caring mother and wife ensuring the comfort and growth of their family. That said, I would not give up my career for anything and am happy that I made that choice, even though it was the harder way.

"The worst thing to do is to make a woman into a man."

Dr. Katalin Nagy

As a woman, I don't want to be like a man. I firmly dislike the idea. I believe that it's important to retain our femininity and all the emotions and sensations that come with our feminine nature. If I were to lose that, then it would feel like a defeat. I don't like women who act like men, as that can make them appear tough, but it's important to stay true to oneself, as a woman. I need to feel good in my own skin on a daily basis and embrace my femininity.

By that, I mean that women are delicate, not weak. Women have different needs and that is natural. It is now proven that women are as efficient at the task, the numbers will back me up on that. So why are we still struggling to admit that our profession needs to adapt? The reality is, and will always be, that a mother will not sleep until her children are sleeping. That is not favour nor special treatment, just the recognition of a reality.

When I was in Colombia, I experienced something that made me feel fantastic. The Latin culture is different when approaching the men-women relationships compared to the United States. In the US, if someone compliments you and asks you out for coffee, they may face legal consequences, but in the Latin world, it's completely normal. I loved it and would love to experience it again.

It is important to feel desired, pretty, and empowered. There is nothing wrong with that! Everybody needs to be reminded of their values, men and women alike! And that is a challenge within our profession, one in which most interactions have been dehumanized and sterilized.

I believe that relationships are becoming very impersonal and I don't like it. I felt good in Colombia and I think that I need to go back there. The freedom to express oneself as a woman is important and I don't want to lose that.

I don't have the answer to how a woman should stand in our profession. But I surely know that embracing our femininity and not denying our nature is the right place to start.

"To have support is not weakness, it is wisdom. To be delicate and kind is our nature. Well, I will even say that it is part of our beauty."

Dr. Katalin Nagy

We should embrace what we are and allow ourselves to feel good about our femininity to, in turn, care for our patients, staff, and colleagues with our gentle touch and kindness.

I was the founder and first Dean of the Faculty of Dentistry at the University of Szeged. I served as dean for 8 years. I was a strong figure of leadership and yet, how many times students and teachers came to my door to express their doubts and challenges? I can't count the number of times where they were crying on my shoulder. Once the tears swept, we could resume our tasks, even with better efficiency.

Our faculty is a family. I went to weddings, and birthdays, and often visited them (teachers and former students) at their homes. Some, have shared meals at my home. I am proud to say that I brought my feminine touch into my work, with warmth, beauty, and kindness.

This is **LEADERSHIP volume 1, CHANGING THE WORLD FROM A DENTAL CHAIR** presented by ALPHA DENTISTRY. Welcome to the Alphas.

Dr. BAK NGUYEN

CHAPTER 13
"THE EDUCATION SYSTEM"
THE COVID GENERATION

Interview of Dr. KATALIN NAGY

Written by Dr. BAK NGUYEN

Establishing new relationships has become quite challenging these days, especially in the US and Europe, including England. Men seem to be hesitant to start a new relationship. I think the situation could be improved if the communication between people was a little bit more relaxed and open. And that is what I truly believe: it should start, with genuine communication to establish a strong relationship amongst peers, amongst colleagues, amongst teachers and students.

I had a few people over at my house yesterday and we discussed this issue and they all shared the same view that we need to ease up on the communication barriers. We had communication challenges prior to COVID. Now, after 2 years of COVID, communication issues are in even worse shape!

The feeling amongst students is that they can date, but there is still an awkwardness in their interactions. As the Dean of the faculty for 8 years, I saw this evolve. During that time, students and colleagues would come to my office and open up to me about their personal and professional problems. Many students even cried on my shoulder about relationship issues.

Although it took a lot of time away from my professional life, the whole faculty felt like a big family and no one wanted to leave. This close bond between students, teachers, and staff was not possible in larger faculties like in the USA. As an educator, it's important to have a unique personality and to incorporate it into our teaching style, not just in the classroom, but outside of it as well. I never asked about students' relationships in class, but after class, I was involved in their personal lives and even was invited to their weddings and birthdays.

We are talking about dating, but relationships are so much broader than love. It is about how 2 individuals interacting with one another, how the individual links built up as pillars of a group dynamic, which in turn are the pillars of how patients and the exterior world perceive us, as a group, as a team and, consequently, as a profession. To bring it down to dating makes it simpler to address but relationship as a broad topic is essential.

And that is where I believe we got lost in translation, making sure to have rules around the dating relationships, of what is allowed and what is not, that we lost sight of how to communicate and forge relationships (non-romantic ones). Look in your books and rules, we know a lot about what NOT to do, but less and less about how to approach relationship and communication and how to apply it in our reality.

"I believe that education is not just about reading books or slides, it's also about bringing in your own personality."

Dr. Katalin Nagy

If you can't give that to your students, you are generic and can be easily replaced. No one won't remember you because they all have access to the information they need online. As a professor and an educator, don't be afraid to build with your personality, philosophy, and what makes you unique as an individual.

As a former Dean of a dental faculty for eight years, I had a lot of interactions with students and colleagues. They would come to me with their personal and professional problems, which took up a lot of my time but also allowed me to bond with the faculty members, who felt like a big family.

"To make an impact, one needs to add their own personality and experiences to the education."

Dr. Katalin Nagy

I introduced a subject called "Communication in Dentistry" into the curriculum which was very well received by the students. We even did role-playing practices and made videos of the students communicating with a patient (played by an actor) to discuss what worked well and what didn't. Although this subject is no longer taught due to a lack of actors and students' interest, I still believe it was an important part of their educational journey. Both parties benefited from that experience, students and educators.

The students showed little interest in a course on communication and human interaction. However, if we examine the facts, our profession is grappling with depression and a shortage of human interactions, despite appearing successful on the surface. It feels like we're on a small ship, adrift and alone.

During the COVID-19 pandemic, students faced many difficulties. Although they did not suffer from the illness itself, they were required to participate in COVID testing and treatment. This made it challenging for them to continue their studies normally. The situation led to a feeling of lethargy amongst students and educators alike.

As a result, the education system became less rigorous, and students learnt that they could receive a diploma with less effort. This has led to a new generation of students who are more laid-back in their approach to education. They are often late for class and are less motivated to attend in person. Educators have also become more relaxed, often opting to hold classes online.

"Some subjects, such as dentistry, cannot be effectively taught online."
Dr. Katalin Nagy

This situation has resulted in a new learning experience for students, as they have realized that they can receive a diploma without putting in as much effort as before.

My observations are that we are already lacking behind in communication skills prior to COVID, focusing on the surgical skills. Now, post-COVID, even the teaching of surgical skills got affected and deemed acceptable. I am worried about this trend and how to counter the lowering of our standards.

My hope is that COVID has caused only temporary damage to our educational system and that we will eventually return to normal. However, I still sense the lingering negative impacts of COVID. Additionally, there is a fear that every time there is news of a COVID wave in China, we may have to shut down again...

I hope that this never happens, as it could lead to the downfall of our dental education system if we have to close down repeatedly.

This is **LEADERSHIP volume 1, CHANGING THE WORLD FROM A DENTAL CHAIR** presented by ALPHA DENTISTRY. Welcome to the Alphas.

Dr. BAK NGUYEN

CHAPTER 14
"CONTINUOUS EDUCATION"
Interview of Dr. KATALIN NAGY

Written by Dr. BAK NGUYEN

I want to emphasize the importance of Masha's postgraduate education program and offer my support. However, the current scale of the program, with only 50 to 100 participants, is not enough. I have been involved in this field for 16 years, and my own program reaches 800 people. The connection to a university is what makes it a full-fledged education system, not just a course.

Inviting guest speakers, even if they are well-known, is not enough if the audience is small. Some speakers charge $10,000 for a 45-minute lecture, and while I also invite these speakers, I allow all university students from Hungary to attend for free. This gives them a unique opportunity to see these prominent figures in person, and it will be a memory they will cherish and share as they go on to work in different parts of the world. To me, that is leadership!

Preparing for a conference like those takes a year in preparation and requires finding sponsors to finance the event and to pay the speakers. The university can't pay for it, so I have to dig into my personal connections.

"To make an impact, one needs to add their own personality and experiences to education."

Dr. Katalin Nagy

That is an example of what I meant when I referred to bringing our personality to education. I leveraged my reputation and the relationships that I built over the years to interest sponsors who will benefit from the exposure of these events. Sponsors are happy to give their support because they know that all the university students will be there, listening and connecting their company name with their education, I made them into partners. This is why having a connection with the university is so important to sponsors, because it officially recognizes the event and its prestige.

I'm trying to maintain a balanced budget and I don't aim for any profit as there's already very little to begin with. Despite treating the guests like royalty with all the dinners and events, we don't end up making much. I spend at least three hours a day working on the conference, handling around 80 emails, and dealing with all the speakers, who only communicate with me and not the sponsoring companies.

The idea of leveraging technology to give the event a second or third life, can be a great idea. A colleague of mine recently suggested that I should record the events or write articles or books about them to increase the prestige of the conference. I don't seek recognition or fame, I just want to continue hosting these events for as long as I can.

I am organizing these dental events for dentists, for my former students, and for all the future dentists of Hungary. I am also doing this, leading by example to inspire other leaders to emerge and to do the same. The world is a big place and we have members of dentistry on all 5 continents. I like to see myself as a part of something much bigger.

"My philosophy, from the beginning, is to share, to empower, and to inspire."
Dr. Katalin Nagy

For the past 2 years, we have been recording videos and taking reports with the speakers on-site during the conference. Previously, there was no documentation of the event. We would edit a small film and play it a few times, but that was it. I have to admit, I'm not very skilled with technology and never thought of the potential benefits of documenting the event in a more impactful way.

In the educational field, many people lack access to resources and opportunities, not just in the field of dentistry, but in many areas. For example, I have been to Nigeria twice and observed the lack of access to conferences or educational systems. This is where videos or online resources could be really helpful, providing educational opportunities to people in these countries.

African countries and many others in Asia can benefit greatly from leveraging technology in education. However, the necessary infrastructure and technical support must be in place in order to bring these ideas to fruition.

Instead of just saying thank you to our sponsors, we could offer them even more. If they are willing to pay a bit more, we can provide them with exposure not just to 800 or 1000 professionals, but to 5 countries. This would require a bit more investment, but if they can afford it, they would become a superpower and their name would be known to many. A friend of mine, who is the President of the Chinese Dental Association, visited me at my home and he expressed that any type of education we can provide to China will be appreciated. There is a high demand for it in the country.

Those are the opportunities that COVID brought to our doors, the chance to network and to share our means at a much broader scope. And to do so, we must master technology and the new means of communication. As for the COVID graduates, they could only benefit from such endeavours, because now, we are talking their language, through a screen and from miles apart! COVID did not just bring bad things but also the opportunity to see our profession globally.

Now, it is an opportunity but not a free giveaway. We would need leaders and passionate members to pick up the torch and to lead the way into the Information Age, to borrow from my friend, Dr. Bak.

As much as I believe that dentistry cannot be taught online, I am also very open to the opportunity for continuous education to step up its scale and scope to reach a global audience.

This is **LEADERSHIP volume 1, CHANGING THE WORLD FROM A DENTAL CHAIR** presented by ALPHA DENTISTRY. Welcome to the Alphas.

Dr. BAK NGUYEN

CHAPTER 15
"THE POSITIVE SIDE OF COVID"
THE OPPORTUNITIES AND THE CHALLENGES
Interview of Dr. KATALIN NAGY

Written by Dr. BAK NGUYEN

While it's true that COVID has had negative effects, it's important to also focus on the positive aspects. One positive aspect is the increased connectivity we've experienced due to the pandemic. I would never have met someone like Masha or Bak if it wasn't for COVID, and now we're the best of friends, both online and in person.

I've also had the opportunity to connect with several big educators and lecturers in the field of dental education, including Alessandro Pozzi, Miguel Stanley, and others. In fact, some of them have become my Ph.D. students, which has allowed us to collaborate on postgraduate courses and research projects. The majority of my experiences have been positive.

During the lockdowns, we had more time to delve into research and work on projects together, and this has led to some great outcomes. Overall, I believe that the impact of COVID on the dental education has been a mixed bag, but there have certainly been some positive aspects that have emerged.

Dental education encompasses not only graduate education but also postgraduate programs as well. Postgraduate education consists of both postgraduate courses and personal education. For example, Masha and I are involved in attending conferences and conducting PTSD research with our students.

These students came to Hungary to collaborate with us, write articles, and do research. I believe that the COVID-19 pandemic gave us a little more time to focus on research because we were in lockdown at the time. And during the lockdown, we were able to focus more on research as we couldn't perform any treatments on patients as it was risky. We took advantage of this time to focus more on research, which is reflected in the increased number of articles we published during and after COVID.

Additionally, the lockdown also provided us with an opportunity to connect with dentists internationally, which would not have been possible otherwise. The use of Zoom calls allowed us to build international connections and interact with people from all over the world. This was a great opportunity to meet new people and exchange ideas, which had never happened before in the dental education field.

In other words, COVID brought us closer as a profession, especially at the leadership level. We should hold on to that. Through a Zoom call, it is now acceptable to collaborate across countries and continents. If there is a chance to seize, it is to hold on to the international connectivity that COVID brought to the table.

To be honest, COVID had both positive and negative impacts on us. I hope we can continue to focus on the positive aspects and build upon them. I believe that international connections are crucial in our field, especially for small countries like Hungary with a unique language. Without these connections, we won't be able to progress on our own.

On the matter of language, the situation in Hungary with regards to language is a bit complicated. English is not widely spoken, and for many years, Russian was the mandatory language, so not everyone had the opportunity to learn other languages. This can make it challenging for professionals in Hungary to make international connections, by extension, to be open to the world outside of our borders.

However, COVID-19 provided a unique opportunity for people in Hungary to connect with others from around the world without leaving their homes or institutions. This was especially beneficial for those who are able to understand English.

It's important to keep these real human interactions and not just rely on virtual communication. Just like I believe that a woman should never try to be a man, I believe in the warmth of human connection and the strength of genuine relationship.

Hosting and inviting people is crucial, as Hungary is known for being a great host. Without these efforts, the connections will not be maintained and the opportunities provided by COVID, lost. In a way, COVID gave us an opportunity to connect with people from different parts of the world with whom we might not have met otherwise. But it's up to us to use this opportunity and not just let it pass by. Some people are satisfied just with online interactions, but others want in-person experiences. If we don't use the opportunities provided by the pandemic, such as Zoom, then we won't benefit from it.

However, if we continue to invite others and show them what we are doing, even if they are not speaking at our conference, we can use this time to our advantage. It's possible to gain something from this lockdown if we continue to leverage the opportunities it has given us.

I started this book talking about balance. Well, this should be a new challenge: to balance, to keep being open to international connections through technology while shaking hands and embracing colleagues in person. I am looking forward to see how we will balance this one.

This is **LEADERSHIP volume 1, CHANGING THE WORLD FROM A DENTAL CHAIR** presented by ALPHA DENTISTRY. Welcome to the Alphas.

Dr. BAK NGUYEN

PART 3

THE LEADS

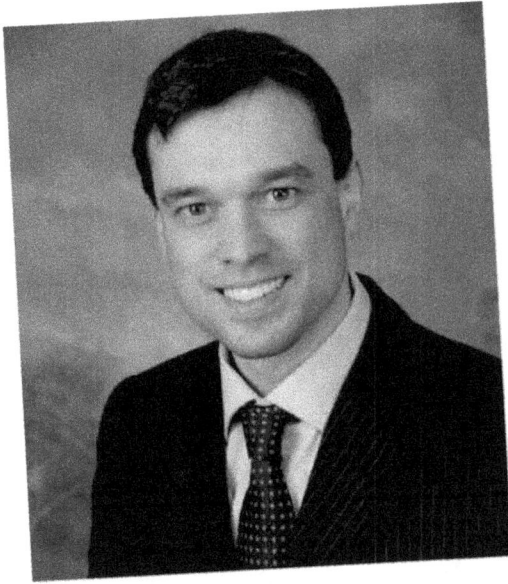

Dr. PAUL DOMINIQUE,
DDS, MS

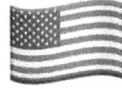

From the USA 🇺🇸, **Dr. & Prof. PAUL DOMINIQUE** is a paediatric dentist, entrepreneur and investor. He's a graduate of the National University of Ireland, where he earned a Bachelor of Science degree in cell biology and molecular genetics. He completed his dental degree at the University of Kentucky and his specialty training in paediatrics at the Eastman Institute for Oral Health, University of Rochester, NY. Dr. Dominique served as an assistant professor in public health at the University of Kentucky, division of oral health science. During his tenure, he headed and improved a novel mobile program that successfully addresses access to care issues for children in Central and Western Kentucky.

Dr. Dominique is also an entrepreneur having acquired and consolidated a small group of practices growing from less than 700K to over 2.4 Million EBITDA in under 24 months. Dr. Dominique has been angel investing for the past decade, investing across a diverse group of platforms such as equity crowdfunding, psychedelic medicine, real estate and teledentistry. He currently serves as a board advisory member to the Teledentists and Revere Partners, the first venture fund dedicated to oral health. He's currently involved in a project that is exploring the use of blockchain technology and NFTs to help improve access to dental care. Dr. Dominique joined the Alphas in 2020 as he contributed to the Teledentistry Summit at the beginning of the COVID crisis. Since Dr. Dominique has contributed to many Alphas summits and books including RELEVANCY and the ALPHA DENTISTRY book franchise (volumes 1 and 4).

CHAPTER 16
"BLOCKCHAIN TECHNOLOGY"
THE SHIFT IN TECHNOLOGY

Interview with Dr. PAUL DOMINIQUE

written by Dr. BAK NGUYEN

Dr. Paul Dominique is a well-respected paediatric dentist, investor, and entrepreneur with a passion for transforming the dental industry. With a focus on making dental care more affordable and disrupting the current status quo, Dr. Dominique is dedicated to ensuring everyone has access to quality preventative dental care, reducing the need for costly restorative and surgical procedures.

Based in the United States, where dental care is amongst the most advanced and accessible in the world, Dr. Dominique is acutely aware of the issue of underutilization of dental services, with around half of the U.S. population not visiting the dentist regularly. He believes that this is not just a problem in the United States, but a global issue that must be addressed. With his strong vision for the future of dentistry, Dr. Dominique is committed to driving positive change in the industry and improving the overall health and well-being of his patients.

STATUS QUO

Access to dental care is a major issue for billions of people around the world. According to statistical research published by Marco Vujicic, the Chief Economist of the American Dental Association and Head of the Health Policy Institute of the American Dental Association, financial barriers are one of the primary reasons why people, in the U.S. find it difficult to access dental care as compared to other forms of healthcare including psychiatric or pharmaceutical care.

The World Health Organization recently published an article titled "The State of Oral Health in the World," which estimates that half of the world's population is affected by some form of oral disease. This is a widespread problem that requires us to leverage advanced technology as manpower alone cannot solve it. It is simply not feasible to train sufficient dentists or auxiliary providers to address the dental care needs of billions of people around the world.

According to a survey by DHM Research, only one-third of Americans have a plan for their life, indicating a lack of foresight and preparedness in certain areas of life, including healthcare. Oral health is a significant aspect of healthcare that requires planning and access to dental care professionals. In the United States, the market capitalization and the utilization of dentistry appear to be increasing, on average every year, however, this "apparent" increase in both of these metrics is actually quite misleading.

The primary reason for the increase in these two metrics is because of the dramatic rise in paediatric utilization, which is heavily (federal) government-subsidized via Medicaid. Another reason is also the rise in utilization among the wealthy older adults of the baby boomer generation with represents most of the expenditure in U.S. dentistry. The combination of the increase in utilization by these two cohorts is masking the real picture which is one of decline for the rest of the population, particularly younger adults (ages 19-46) for which this decline goes back to 1997.

As stated earlier, in the U.S., dentistry is the most advanced and accessible in the world. If the rates of utilization are already subpar in the U.S. one can only imagine how much worse there are elsewhere.

In the late 1990s, the U.S. government solidified their support for paediatric dentistry via the Medicaid system. This came after national media attention of an African American child named Diamante Driver who died of a brain abscess caused by an abscessed tooth. Today (data from 2021) U.S. federal government support for dentistry tops USD 25 Billion more than the GDP of the island nation of Jamaica. Therefore, it's not hard to extrapolate that most countries in the world have very limited utilization.

The decline in dental visits by younger adults is concerning, as this age group represents a significant cohort of the population. As a result, the government acknowledges that children are a vulnerable population who do not have a choice in selecting their parents and has since been expanding and trying to make dentistry more accessible for low-income families and children.

The government-sponsored Children's Dental Service is responsible for the increase in market capitalization in dentistry, but it is also masking the decreasing rate of the number of younger adults visiting the dentist.

In addition to the younger adults' decline, access to dental care is also declining amongst the adult population who do not have government-sponsored dental care, indicating a potential issue with affordability or insurance coverage. Given that this decline is happening in the United States, it is likely occurring in other countries as well, potentially to a greater extent. Therefore, the major problem in dental care is access to care, particularly for vulnerable populations such as children and low-income families.

As a response, the Canadian government recently voted a universal dental coverage to include most part of its population to have access to dental care.

SOCIO-ECONOMY

One significant barrier is the shortage of dental health professionals in many areas, which affects 53 million Americans who have limited access to dental care. The number of dentists per 100,000 population is highest in Washington D.C. (103) and lowest in South-Eastern United States (45 per 100,000), with the national average being 61. In addition to the shortage of dental health professionals, there are also issues with healthcare affordability and access.

About 1 in 10 people in the United States do not have health insurance, and people without insurance are less likely to have a primary care provider, which can affect access to dental care services and medications they need.

In fact, according to statistics, only 64% of U.S. adults aged 18 to 64 years stated they had a dental visit in the past 12 months in 2020. This percentage varies by income, with those earning less having less access to dental care. Furthermore, dental emergencies can be a significant burden on the healthcare system and access to preventative dental care can help reduce the number of emergency room visits.

In addition, the current modus operandi of two dental cleanings per year does not suffice. Instead, a more ad hoc system of dental prophylaxis that determines dental cleanings based on the condition of the patient's mouth needs to be adopted. This system would entail more frequent cleanings that would be determined by conditions in the patient's mouth.

For instance, an average woman in the industrialized world gets her hair and nails done every month but only goes to the dentist twice a year. Older populations tend to maintain a good quality of care for their front teeth, which are more visible, but not for their back teeth, which require more manual dexterity to clean.

TECHNOLOGY AS A SOLUTION

The proposed technological solution involves employing teledentistry, artificial intelligence, web 3.0, and blockchain. Teledentistry refers to the use of telecommunication technology to provide dental care from a distance. Artificial intelligence can be used to perform virtual dental examinations and analyze patient data to identify the state of their oral health. Web 3.0 technology can be used to create decentralized systems that enable the secure sharing of dental health data.

Blockchain technology can also be employed to **incentivize** patients to share their oral data with dental care providers in a timely manner to intervene before dental problems become expensive to treat.

TELE-DENTISTRY

The statistics on dental-related emergency room visits in the US are staggering. According to data from 2017, US hospitals billed $2.7 billion for dental-related emergency room visits, while Pacific Dental Service, the largest Dental Support Organization (DSO) in the world, billed $1.3 billion in revenue during the same year.

This means that the combined billing of US hospitals for dental emergencies where patients saw a physician instead of a dentist was more than double the revenue of the largest dental corporation in the world. This highlights the need for dentists to find better solutions to prevent dental emergencies and to provide more cost-effective care to patients. One potential solution to this crisis in dentistry is tele-dentistry.

Tele-dentistry is the use of interactive audio, video, data communications, and other tele-health systems to provide and support dental care delivery, diagnosis, consultation, treatment, transfer of dental information, and education. The American Dental Association has provided interim guidance on coding and billing for tele-dentistry services during the COVID-19 pandemic.

Tele-dentistry has the potential to increase access to care, enhance the patient experience, improve health outcomes, and reduce costs for both patients and dentists. While the use of consults by dentists in emergency rooms is a step in the right direction, there is still more that can be done to prevent dental problems from happening in the first place.

Leveraging technology and innovation can help to prevent dental emergencies and reduce costs for patients and dentists. Tele-dentistry is a promising solution that can help to provide preventive care and early intervention for dental problems. By using tele-dentistry, dentists can remotely monitor patients and provide early intervention for dental problems, reducing the need for costly emergency room visits.

The crisis in dentistry requires a shift towards preventive care and cost-effective solutions. Tele-dentistry has the potential to provide increased access to care, enhance the patient experience, improve health outcomes, and reduce costs for both patients and dentists. While it may not be a complete solution, tele-dentistry can play a significant role in addressing the crisis in dentistry and providing better care for patients.

BLOCKCHAIN TECHNOLOGY

As a paediatric dentist and Medicaid provider, our dental practices see a high volume of patients, and we have developed efficient techniques due to our low reimbursement rates. We have mastered the flow of efficiently cleaning patients' mouths, including adolescents and teenagers with braces, in a timely manner. This is achieved by having high-volume production with a lot of space and auxiliaries to assist in moving patients through clinics.

The solution to making dental care more accessible is to offer dental cleanings at a nominal price or subscription fee while leveraging technology such as AI, which is continually improving as it is trained on more data. With frequent virtual examinations, live dentists may not be necessary for every patient as AI can accurately calculate a patient's plaque score at any given moment.

This technology can be built on blockchain, ensuring efficiency and automation where human intervention is only necessary for complex cases or auditing purposes to maintain quality assurance. Blockchain technology has become increasingly relevant in the healthcare industry, including in dental care.

As a ledger in dental software, blockchain allows for secure storage, time-stamping, and easy accessibility of patient records. Patients can also use blockchain to tokenize their oral cavity, which allows them to leverage their data as an asset for monetary gain. For example, a patient can use their 3D scan to entice a dentist to recruit them as a patient.

Additionally, blockchain features such as smart contracts automate contracts on the blockchain, eliminating the need for human oversight. However, with the increased availability of patient data comes concerns about privacy. Blockchain technology offers a unique solution to this problem. Patients are in full control of their data, and they can choose with whom they want to share it.

This is in contrast to Web 2.0, where individuals often cede control of their data to technology companies such as Facebook and Google, which monetize and sell that data. In essence, blockchain technology represents a shift in the balance of power from large technology companies to individuals.

The individual now has control over their data and can use them to their advantage in ways that were previously unavailable. The potential benefits of blockchain in healthcare are significant, and its use in dental care is just one example of how this technology can revolutionize the industry.

A NEW ECONOMIC MODEL

Many people avoid going to the dentist due to financial constraints, and blockchain technology offers a potential solution to this problem. Through blockchain, patients can tokenize their oral cavity, turning what was once a liability into an asset.

Patients can digitize their dental records, making them easily accessible to dentists who can search for patients they want to treat. Blockchain technology also provides patients with full control over their data, allowing them to monetize it and decide whom they want to share it with.

Dentists can leverage blockchain to keep a record of everything they do with their patients, making patient records easily accessible and time-stamped. Blockchain also allows for fully automated smart contracts, eliminating the need for human oversight. Blockchain technology can change the dental industry by allowing dentists to access a database of digitized oral cavities created by patients and pay to access that data.

This allows dentists to cherry-pick the patients they want to work with and pay patients to access their data to recruit those patients, making the entire process more efficient and cost-effective. Additionally, companies that aggregate patients' health data, including dental data, are likely to become the next billion-dollar companies, driving innovation and growth in the healthcare sector.

In the future, wearable technology will play a significant role in gathering health data from patients. Devices that patients can put in their mouths to monitor biofilm already exist, and AI can detect biofilm, allowing patients to effectively manage dental disease.

By monitoring patients' biofilm on a regular basis, dentists can combine that data with professional cleanings to manage dental diseases more effectively and lower the cost of dental care for the population. The crisis in the dental profession has persisted for the past 2 decades or more. This problem cannot be solved through manpower alone.

Instead, we need to leverage technology. The boards of dentistry and the provinces in both Canada and the United States need to adapt to changes in the field. Currently, the buzzwords in medicine revolve around analytical-based reimbursement and outcomes-based reimbursement, as opposed to procedural-based reimbursement.

Dentistry is a decade behind in this regard, but we need to catch up. Medicine recognizes the need for change, and patients can now have legitimate medical visits via telemedicine. We are not there yet in dentistry. Leveraging technology like tele-dentistry and blockchain technology provides the potential to revolutionize the healthcare industry, from patient data to treatment options. It solves the financing problem and puts the control back in the hands of patients.

With blockchain technology, patients can monetize their data and dental implant manufacturers can streamline their marketing efforts, passing on the savings to patients. This solution is the beginning of solving the affordability issue of dental care. Blockchain technology offers efficiency in scheduling and staffing needs for dentists, leading to cost savings for patients and a better overall experience. The combination of technology and prevention will be the solution to the dental pandemic silently occurring for decades. This goes beyond dentistry and healthcare.

Wearable technology also has the potential to play a significant role in gathering health data from patients and lowering the cost of dental care for the population. New companies need data, and they need it efficiently.

Web 3.0 technology allows individuals to be rewarded for sharing their data, and we must pay attention to this in dentistry. Otherwise, we will be left behind and spend another decade looking at the same problem.

This is **LEADERSHIP volume 1, CHANGING THE WORLD FROM A DENTAL CHAIR** presented by ALPHA DENTISTRY. Welcome to the Alphas.

Dr. BAK NGUYEN

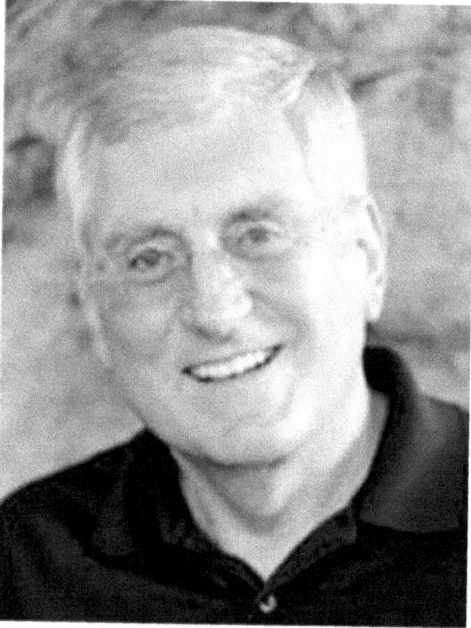

Dr. PAUL OUELLETTE,
DDS, MS, ABO, AFAAID

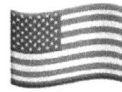

From the USA, **Dr. & Prof. PAUL OUELLETTE**, DDS, MS, ABO, AFAAID, WORLD TOP 100 DOCTOR 2020, Former Associate Professor Georgia School of Orthodontics and Jacksonville University. Highly motivated to help my sons become successful in the "Ouellette Family of Dentists" Group Dental Specialty Practice. During the Pandemic, Dr. Ouellette was amongst the co-founders of the ALPHAS. He also advances his research in the field of mobile dentistry and makes the practice of dentistry affordable and accessible to everyone from everywhere. Dr. Ouellette has contributed to many Alphas summits and books including RELEVANCY, MIDAS TOUCH, THE POWER OF DR, AMONGST THE ALPHAS, KISS ORTHODONTICS and the ALPHA DENTISTRY book franchise.

CHAPTER 17
"MOBILE DENTISTRY"
SAFETY, ACCESSIBILITY, AFFORDABILITY

Interview with Dr. PAUL OUELLETTE

written by Dr. BAK NGUYEN

In the wake of the COVID-19 pandemic, the dental industry has faced significant challenges in providing safe, accessible, and affordable dental services to patients. Dr. Paul Ouellette has developed a mobile dental clinic that addresses these issues on three vectors: **SAFETY**, **ACCESSIBILITY**, and **AFFORDABILITY**.

Dr. Ouellette's mobile clinic is equipped with the latest technology, including active air exchanges and windows, HEPA filtration, and ultraviolet light, to mitigate aerosol contamination during dental procedures. The clinic is designed to be accessible and convenient for seniors, addressing the unique oral health needs of older adults.

Finally, leasing a mobile clinic provides an affordable and flexible solution for dental graduates burdened with student loan debt, allowing them to pursue their desired career paths. With innovative solutions like mobile dentistry, the dental industry can continue to provide high-quality, patient-centred dental care to underserved communities.

Dr. Paul Ouellette, is a highly accomplished orthodontist with over 50 years of experience in the field. He attended Texas A&M for college and Loyola University in Chicago for dental school, where he also completed his orthodontic residency.

After graduation, he began teaching at Emory School of Dentistry before starting his own multiple locations private practices. Over the years, he has owned or been partners in over thirty-three dental locations across several states in the US, and he is still actively involved in multidisciplinary dentistry alongside his two sons, who have also followed in his footsteps. Dr. Ouellette is known for his expertise in orthodontic treatment and has been a pioneer in the use of sonographic imaging. Despite his many accomplishments, Dr. Ouellette is also a humanitarian, philanthropist, author, and inventor who is passionate about implementing cutting-edge dental technology in his practice.

LEADERSHIP

During the COVID-19 pandemic, Dr. Ouellette was concerned about exposure to aerosols in the multidisciplinary practices he was affiliated with. He decided to create a mobile clinic in a sprinter van, but it was too small for dental needs. He then researched cargo trailers and found a company in South Georgia that specialized in outfitting trailers for various medical and dental purposes.

He worked with them to manufacture and outfit two cargo trailers, each with two dental chairs, a digital X-ray machine, full sterilization equipment, suction, and solar backup generators, allowing them to function without being plugged into a building.

Dr. Ouellette has a consortium of partners working with him on his mobile clinic solutions, including orthodontic laboratories. The mobile clinics focus on providing diagnostic triage, a nonprofit service funded through donations and government grants. They offer free triage, cleanings, and fluoride treatments for children and adults and create a comprehensive diagnostic treatment plan for each patient.

Utilizing the newest technologies and safety protocols available, Dr. Ouellette is also looking to store all dental data including X-rays, and photography to be securely stored using blockchain technology in a non-fungible token (NFT). Patients will have control and full ownership of their own data.

SAFETY

The COVID-19 pandemic has created unique challenges for dental organizations worldwide, with open-plan clinics, dental hospitals, and universities experiencing the most significant impacts. One of the most pressing concerns has been the risk of aerosol contamination during dental procedures, which can potentially spread the virus.

While many common dental procedures have a low risk of increasing the aerosol spread of COVID-19, research has shown that efficient airflow engineering, surface disinfection, and air filtration devices can help mitigate aerosol contamination in dental settings.

The Centre for Disease Control and Prevention (CDC) has updated its COVID-19 guidance for dental settings, recommending that dental healthcare personnel should only avoid aerosol-generating dental procedures for patients with suspected or confirmed COVID-19, rather than avoiding aerosol-generating procedures for all patients. The CDC's infection control guidance for COVID-19 includes recommendations on wearing personal protective equipment (PPE) and precautions to follow when performing aerosol-generating procedures.

Despite the low risk of transmission, precautions are necessary to protect patients and staff, including the use of FFP3 masks and extra time between patients to allow aerosol to disperse. The American Dental Association (ADA) conducted a survey which found that 99% of dentists have implemented additional infection prevention and control procedures due to the COVID-19 pandemic. The need to protect dentists and patients and reduce the amount of spatter produced during dental procedures remains a concern, leading to a dramatic reduction in dental services.

In 2020, dental care utilization decreased by 38% compared to 2019, with dental spending decreasing by an estimated $64 billion, according to the American Dental Association. These statistics highlight the significant impact of the pandemic on dental care utilization and spending. So fear has contributed to impact even more an industry already challenged by the general perception of pain and fear. Well, there is a solution and not a too far-fetched one!

Mobile dentistry has emerged as a viable solution to mitigate the impact of the pandemic on dental services. Mobile dental clinics can facilitate the control of aerosols during dental procedures, providing a safe and convenient alternative to traditional dental clinics. They have the advantage of reducing volume since there is no longer a waiting room.

Mobile clinics utilize HEPA filtration and ultraviolet light to treat and quickly turn over the air, ensuring clean air for patients. Dr. Ouellette's mobile clinic is equipped with active air exchanges and windows, making it easier to have complete air exchange with the exterior.

The mobile clinic is designed to allow the patient to undergo the procedure alone, while their parents or guardians stay in their cars. The mobile clinics provide communication with parents and guardians through iPhone apps and stream video from inside the clinic, allowing them to see what's happening and communicate with the dental professionals as necessary.

As soon as the procedure is over, a staff member accompanies the child back to their parents while the room is getting disinfected and the air is completely purged with the exterior air. And what about the environment and global warming issues? While mobile clinics require driving, the solution is a trailer to be pulled by a conventional car. The impact of mobile clinics on air quality and carbon footprint can be mitigated by using electric vehicles in the future.

Mobile clinics can visit underserved neighbourhoods, prisons, and physical locations, and patients can wait in their cars or nearby building waiting rooms. In that sense, bringing the service to the people may help to decrease travelling and contribute to the green effort while making the experience safer for all patients.

ACCESSIBILITY
PROBLEM 2: SENIORS

The ongoing COVID-19 pandemic has presented unique challenges for the dental field in North America, particularly in providing services to senior people who are at a higher risk of severe illness or death from the virus. In addition to ensuring their safety during dental appointments, dental providers must also address the unique oral health needs of older adults who are more likely to experience tooth decay, gum disease, tooth loss, and other age-related oral health issues.

To address these challenges, dental providers must implement additional infection control measures, such as the use of personal protective equipment, screening protocols, and enhanced cleaning and disinfection procedures. It is also crucial for dental providers to have a thorough understanding of the health status and medical history of their older adult patients to effectively address their oral health needs.

Access to dental care is another significant challenge for senior people in North America, as many older adults may have limited mobility or transportation, making it difficult for them to travel to a dental clinic. Furthermore, dental care can be unaffordable or financially challenging for those living on a fixed income. Innovative solutions such as mobile dental clinics combined with tele-dentistry services delivered in the patient's home can address these barriers to care.

The mobile clinics are designed to be accessible and convenient for seniors in retirement homes, with an ADA certified wheelchair ramp and a motorized awning that provides shade and shelter for patients. It features two dental chairs equipped with an X-ray machine and an intraoral scanners that eliminate the need for messy impressions.

The use of 3D printing technology in dentistry is another innovative solution that can address the challenges faced by senior people in North America which is built into Dr. Ouellette's mobile solution.

3D printing technology enables the creation of various dental parts, including aligners, dentures, and crowns, with exceptional precision and accuracy. This technology allows for the customization of dental appliances that match the patient's anatomy and provide greater comfort. Furthermore, the production of 3D-printed dentures is considerably less expensive than traditional dentures.

The mobile clinic also utilizes 3D printing technology to produce cost-effective and fast digital dentistry solutions, including surgical guides for implants and provisional dentures. These solutions can significantly improve the quality of life for seniors, helping them to eat and function better, feel better about themselves, and boost their overall well-being and self-esteem.

Mobile clinics offer a safer, more flexible, and more cost-effective option for providing dental services to underserved communities. With the right protocols and workflows in place, mobile clinics can be a valuable addition to the dental industry.

AFFORDABILITY
PROBLEM 3: DENTAL GRADUATES

The cost of tuition and student loan debt for dental graduates in the United States has been a major issue for many years. According to the American Dental Education Association, the average debt per dental school graduate in 2020 was around $301,000 to $304,000.

This significant amount of debt poses several challenges for new dentists, such as affecting their career choices and personal finances. Late student loan payments can negatively impact a dentist's credit score, making it challenging for them to obtain financing for significant purchases like a home or car.

Although the COVID-19 pandemic has had some impact on student loan debt for dental school graduates, the CARES Act has temporarily set interest rates on all federally-owned loans, including Direct Loans used to finance dental school education, at 0%. However, managing student loan debt effectively remains crucial for maintaining a strong credit score and financial stability.

This high level of debt makes it challenging for new graduates to choose their preferred career path and may affect their ability to secure financing for opening their own clinic or purchasing an existing practice. Other challenges may include finding employment opportunities in the desired location or field of dentistry, obtaining necessary certifications, and managing the financial and administrative aspects of running a dental practice.

The high cost of tuition and the level of debt associated with it serve as significant obstacles for those seeking to open their clinics. This high level of debt makes it challenging for graduates to borrow more money to invest in their own practice. Opening a new dental clinic requires a substantial investment in equipment and facilities, which can be challenging to fund with such a high level of debt. As a result, many dental graduates opt to work for established practices instead of starting their clinics.

To help dentists overcome these challenges, leasing a mobile clinic could be a great alternative solution. As a lease, it is affordable and accessible to all dentists, even new graduates. This solution provides a flexible solution to modernize equipment (renewed every 5 years).

The credit score and debt ratio are less demanding on a lease than on a conventional mortgage. Keep in mind that the comparison will be to have a bricks and mortars clinic with a minimal cost of $500,000, which, at 7% interest and amortized over 10 years, represents a monthly payment of $5,805 plus taxes, and the rent is to be added on top of that.

Depending on the equipment requirement, Dr. Ouellette's mobile clinics are ranging between $3000 to $5000 a month. Considering the rent factor of another $3000 to $5000 a month in the case of conventional bricks and mortars clinics, dentists are looking at a saving of at least 50% of their related expenses.

In addition, leasing a mobile clinic is safer and upgradeable, and it can be updated every 5 years, while also opening up new markets, such as senior care and school service. This mobile solution is surely a great alternative for dentists to help them overcome their financial challenges and pursue their desired career paths.

The dental industry faces significant challenges related to safety, accessibility, and affordability, particularly in the wake of the COVID-19 pandemic. However, innovative solutions such as mobile dental clinics and tele-dentistry services, combined with 3D printing technology and affordable leasing options, can help overcome these challenges and provide safer, more flexible, and more cost-effective dental care to underserved communities, including seniors and new dental graduates.

By leveraging technology and adopting new business models, the dental industry can continue to provide high-quality care while addressing the unique needs of patients and dental professionals alike.

This is **LEADERSHIP volume 1, CHANGING THE WORLD FROM A DENTAL CHAIR** presented by ALPHA DENTISTRY. Welcome to the Alphas.

Dr. BAK NGUYEN

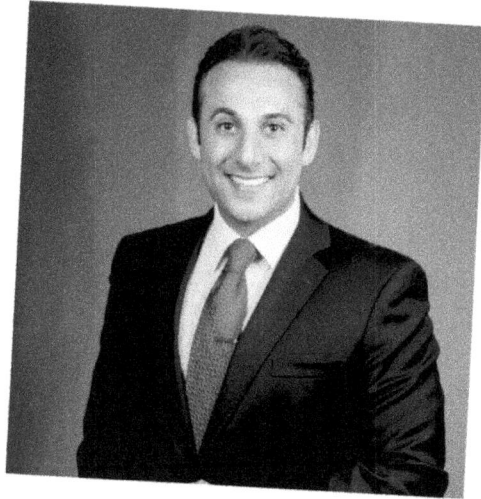

Dr. ARASH HAKHAMIAN,
DDS

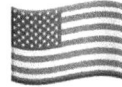

From the USA 🇺🇸, **Dr. ARASH HAKHAMIAN**, DDS, is a leading expert in teledentistry, with over a decade of experience in the field. He is the founder and CEO of Dentulu, the world's leading teledentistry company which was awarded the Best Teledentistry Technology two times at the American Dental Association. Dr. Hakhamian has dedicated his career to improving access to high-quality dental care through the use of technology, and he is a strong advocate for the use of teledentistry to improve patient outcomes and increase accessibility to dental care. As the CEO of Dentulu, Dr. Hakhamian has helped to revolutionize the field of teledentistry, developing innovative technologies and services that enable dental professionals to provide care remotely. Dentulu's platform provides patients with access to a wide range of dental services, including virtual consultations, at-home dental exams, and remote monitoring. With Dentulu, patients can receive high-quality dental care from the comfort of their own homes, reducing the need for travel and time off work. Dr. Hakhamian's approach to Teledentistry exceeds traditional video conferencing and utilizes at-home impression kits to enable the delivery of actual dental services such as sleep apnea devices, mouth-guards, and tooth replacement.

Dr. Hakhamian is a strong advocate for the use of teledentistry to improve patient engagement, convenience, and affordability. He believes that teledentistry has the potential to transform the way dental care is delivered, making it more accessible, affordable, and convenient for patients. Dr. Hakhamian is committed to continuing to innovate and drive the field of teledentistry forward, ensuring that patients around the world have access to high-quality dental care, regardless of their location or financial resources.In this book, Dr. Hakhamian will share his expertise in teledentistry, discussing the latest trends, technologies, and best practices for providing dental care remotely. His insights will be invaluable to dental professionals, patients, and anyone interested in the future of dental care.

CHAPTER 18

"TELE-DENTISTRY"

THE FUTURE WITHIN REACH

By Dr. ARASH HAKHAMIAN

Tele-dentistry is a relatively new approach to dental care, enabled by the rapid advancements in technology in recent years. The term "tele-dentistry" refers to the use of telecommunication technologies to provide dental care remotely. This includes the use of video conferencing, store-and-forward technology, and remote patient monitoring, among other approaches.

The concept of tele-dentistry has been around for several decades, but it wasn't until the advent of high-speed internet and the development of high-quality intraoral cameras that the field began to take off. In the early days of tele-dentistry, dental professionals relied on low-resolution cameras and basic teleconferencing tools to provide remote consultations and follow-up appointments.

However, as technology continued to evolve, so did tele-dentistry. Today, dental professionals can provide a wide range of services remotely, including consultations, diagnoses, treatment planning, and even some types of procedures. The use of personal intraoral cameras, augmented reality, Artificial Intelligence, and other advanced technologies have made it possible for dental professionals to provide accurate diagnoses and treatment plans remotely, enhancing the overall quality of care.

Tele-dentistry has also become increasingly popular in recent years, driven by the demand for more convenient and accessible dental care. The COVID-19 pandemic has further accelerated the adoption of tele-dentistry, as dental professionals and patients seek ways to maintain oral health while minimizing the risk of exposure to the virus and to maintain continuity of care even during shutdowns.

In this chapter, we will explore the evolution and history of tele-dentistry, discussing the latest trends, technologies, and best practices for providing dental care remotely. We will also explore the potential benefits of tele-dentistry, including increased patient engagement, convenience, and affordability, and how tele-dentistry is transforming the field of dentistry. This chapter will also explore the limitations of Tele-dentistry and the importance that dental professionals stay engaged in the shaping of how Tele-dentistry is practiced.

BENEFITS OF TELE-DENTISTRY

Tele-dentistry has numerous benefits for patients, including:

1. **ACCESSIBILITY:** Tele-dentistry can help patients in remote or rural areas access dental care that they may not have been able to receive otherwise. With the widespread use of mobile phones, tablets, and computers, patients can access tele-dentistry services from virtually anywhere, without having to travel long distances to see a dental professional. Mobile phones and tablets are particularly useful for tele-dentistry as they are portable and readily available. Patients can use their mobile devices to access virtual consultations, at-home dental exams, and other tele-dentistry services, allowing them to receive dental care from the comfort of their own homes.

   Moreover, tele-dentistry platforms like Dentulu offer patients the ability to upload images of their teeth and gums, enabling dental professionals to remotely assess their oral health and develop a treatment plan. This can be particularly useful for patients who have limited access to transportation or who live in remote areas where there may not be a dental office nearby. In remote or rural areas, there may be a shortage of dental professionals, or patients may have difficulty travelling to a dental office due to transportation issues or other factors. Tele-dentistry can help address these challenges by providing patients with remote access to high-quality dental care.

2.   **CONVENIENCE:** Tele-dentistry allows patients to receive dental care from the comfort of their own homes or workplaces, saving time and travel costs. Tele-dentistry provides an opportunity to increase convenience for both patients and dental professionals. By eliminating the need for in-person consultations and follow-up appointments, tele-dentistry reduces the amount of time patients need to spend travelling to and from dental offices. This can be particularly beneficial for patients who live in remote or rural areas, where access to dental care can be limited. In addition, tele-dentistry allows dental professionals to provide care to patients more efficiently, reducing the need for lengthy in-person appointments and enabling dental professionals to see more patients in less time.

These benefits are not limited to underserved communities. There is a large portion of the population that is fully capable of paying for dental care, has access to dental insurance, and is fully informed of the importance of oral health. The reality remains that over 164 Million work hours or more are lost annually due to dental visits. This results in the underutilization of dental insurance and dental services that are readily available. Tele-dentistry and mobile dentistry have the potential to increase accessibility to convenient dental services that have a broader impact on the general population even beyond underserved areas.

3.   **COST-EFFECTIVENESS:** Tele-dentistry can be less expensive than traditional dental care, particularly for routine check-ups and consultations. Tele-dentistry also has the potential to drive down the cost of dental care, making it more affordable for patients. By eliminating the need for in-person consultations and follow-up appointments, tele-dentistry can reduce the overall cost of dental care. This can be particularly beneficial for patients who do not have dental insurance or who have limited financial resources. In addition, tele-dentistry can reduce the need for expensive equipment and office space, enabling dental professionals to provide care at a lower cost.

Tele-dentistry significantly reduces dental care prices by lowering the overhead costs associated with traditional dental practices. One of the most significant cost savings of tele-dentistry is the reduction of services that are bound to brick-and-mortar dental offices. This reduction in overhead costs can be passed on to patients in the form of lower prices. Additionally, tele-dentistry eliminates the need for patients to travel to dental offices as often, which can be a significant expense for some patients. Moreover, remote patient monitoring can help identify dental issues early on, preventing them from becoming more severe and costly to treat in the future. All of these factors contribute to the overall affordability of tele-dentistry, making it a promising solution for increasing access to dental care and improving oral health outcomes.

4. **IMPROVED PATIENT EDUCATION:** Tele-dentistry can help patients better understand their dental conditions and treatment options through visual aids and interactive communication. Tele-dentistry provides patients access to 3D imaging and augmented reality technology, patient education, real-time biofeedback and other technologies which can help them visualize complex dental procedures and better understand their treatment options. For example, a dental professional can use 3D imaging to show a patient the before-and-after images of their dental restoration procedure, allowing them to see the transformation of their smile in real time.

5. **BETTER COLLABORATION BETWEEN DENTAL PROFESSIONALS:** Tele-dentistry enables dentists and other dental professionals to collaborate more effectively and efficiently, improving patient outcomes. With tele-dentistry, dental professionals can share patient data, images, and treatment plans in real-time, regardless of their location. This can be particularly beneficial for patients who require complex or multi-disciplinary care, as it enables dental professionals from different specialties to collaborate and develop a comprehensive treatment plan.Tele-dentistry also enables dental professionals to share knowledge and expertise, improving the overall quality of care provided. For example, a dental professional who specializes in restorative dentistry can consult with a periodontist to develop a treatment plan for a patient with gum disease and missing teeth.

6. **INCREASED PATIENT ENGAGEMENT:** Tele-dentistry provides an opportunity to increase patient engagement by making dental care more accessible and convenient. Patients are more likely to engage with dental care when it is easy to access and fits into their busy schedules. Tele-dentistry allows patients to receive dental care from the comfort of their own homes, reducing the need for travel and time off work. This convenience factor can be particularly appealing to patients who have mobility issues, live far away from

dental offices, or have busy schedules. The use of interactive technologies, such as Artificial Intelligence and augmented reality, can also increase patient engagement by providing patients with a more personalized and interactive experience. Since most people utilize their mobile phones and computers for a significant portion of the day, reaching them on these devices can prove to be effective and convenient for both patients and providers.

CLASSIFICATION OF TELE DENTISTRY

Tele-dentistry can be classified into different categories based on the type of services provided and the technology used. The five different classifications of tele-dentistry are:

1. **LIVE VIDEO CONFERENCING:** This type of tele-dentistry involves real-time communication between a dental professional and a patient through video conferencing. It can be used for consultations, follow-up appointments, and emergency consultations.

2. **STORE-AND-FORWARD:** Store-and-forward tele-dentistry involves sending patient information, such as

images and diagnostic data, to a dental professional who can review and diagnose the information at a later time. This approach is useful for providing remote consultations and for obtaining second opinions.

3. **REMOTE PATIENT MONITORING:** Remote patient monitoring involves the use of sensors and other technology to monitor a patient's oral health remotely. This type of tele-dentistry is useful for tracking a patient's progress during treatment, such as orthodontic treatment, and for identifying potential issues before they become more serious.

4. **MOBILE HEALTH:** Mobile health tele-dentistry involves the use of mobile devices, such as smartphones and tablets, to provide dental care remotely. This type of tele-dentistry can be used for consultations, remote monitoring, and patient education.

5. **MERGED SERVICES:** This type of tele-dentistry involves combining two or more types of tele-dentistry, such as live video conferencing, remote patient monitoring, at-home impression trays, and delivery of oral appliances directly to patients through Tele-dentistry. This type of tele-dentistry is particularly useful for patients who require

ongoing care, have mobility issues, or do not have dental offices readily available in their area.

MACRO-DRIVERS OF TELEDENTISTRY
UBERIZATION TRENDS DRIVING THE ADVANCEMENT OF TELE-DENTISTRY

Now that we have established Tele-dentistry as a rapidly growing field with the potential to transform the way dental care is delivered, lets discuss some of the external and macro trends driving Tele-dentistry adoption.

While the list is very long, there are several specific trends that are driving the advancement of tele-dentistry and it is important for dental professionals and patients alike to be aware of these trends and their potential impact. Here are some of the most influential macro events in Dentistry driving the adoption of Tele-dentistry:

1. **INCREASING DEMAND FOR CONVENIENT AND ACCESSIBLE DENTAL CARE:** Patients are increasingly seeking dental care that is convenient, accessible, and affordable. Tele-dentistry offers a solution to these challenges by providing patients with the ability to receive dental care remotely, from the comfort of their own homes.

2. **ADVANCEMENTS IN TECHNOLOGY:** Rapid advancements in technology, such as high-quality intraoral cameras, augmented reality, and Artificial Intelligence, are making it possible for dental professionals to provide more accurate diagnoses and treatment plans remotely. This technology is also improving the patient experience, making it easier for patients to access dental care and understand their treatment options.

3. **GROWING ACCEPTANCE OF TELE-DENTISTRY BY DENTAL PROFESSIONALS:** As tele-dentistry becomes more widely accepted and adopted by dental professionals, patients will have greater access to high-quality dental care. Dental professionals are recognizing the potential of tele-dentistry to improve patient outcomes, reduce costs, and enhance the overall quality of care.

4. **INCREASING DEMAND FOR VIRTUAL CONSULTATIONS AND REMOTE MONITORING:** Virtual consultations and remote monitoring are becoming increasingly popular among patients. These services allow patients to receive care without leaving their homes, reducing the need for travel and time off work. Virtual consultations and remote monitoring also enable dental professionals to monitor patient progress and provide timely interventions when

necessary.

5. **IMPACT OF COVID-19 PANDEMIC:** The COVID-19 pandemic has accelerated the adoption of tele-dentistry as dental professionals and patients seek ways to maintain oral health while minimizing the risk of exposure to the virus. The pandemic has highlighted the importance of tele-health and its potential to transform the healthcare industry.

UBERIZATION OF DENTISTRY

I have lectured for many years on the subject of the **UBERIZATION** of Dentistry which is being spearheaded by tele-dentistry. The term **"UBERIZATION"** has become a popular way to describe the transformation of various industries, including the dental industry. The key characteristics of **UBERIZATION** are the use of technology to disrupt traditional industries, the focus on providing on-demand services, and the emphasis on the sharing economy. These characteristics can be applied to tele-dentistry, which is leading the overall **UBERIZATION** of dentistry.

By leveraging cutting-edge technologies such as Artificial Intelligence, augmented reality, and video conferencing, tele-dentistry is changing the way dental care is delivered.

These technologies enable dental professionals to provide remote consultations, at-home dental exams, and other services, providing patients with a more convenient and accessible alternative to traditional dental care.

Another characteristic of **UBERIZATION** is the focus on providing on-demand services. Tele-dentistry platforms such as Dentulu offer patients virtual consultations, at-home dental exams, and remote monitoring, among other services. These platforms enable patients to access dental care from anywhere, at any time, without the need for in-person consultations or follow-up appointments. This on-demand approach to dental care is more convenient for patients, who can access care on their own schedule, and can potentially reduce the overall cost of dental care.

The sharing economy is another key characteristic of **UBERIZATION**, and tele-dentistry fits this model as well. Tele-dentistry platforms like Dentulu provide dental professionals with an opportunity to expand their reach beyond their local community. By providing dental care remotely, dental professionals can see more patients in less time, potentially increasing their revenue and expanding their patient base. This sharing economy approach to dental care is beneficial for both patients and dental professionals.

AT-HOME DENTAL SERVICES

At-home care is a common application of Tele-dentistry. Patients can be sent at-home impression trays to take impressions of their teeth, which can then be sent back to a licensed dental professional for review. This process can be used for a variety of procedures, including the creation of custom-fit dental appliances, such as mouth guards or retainers, and for orthodontic treatments, such as clear aligners. At-home care is particularly useful for patients who have difficulty travelling to a dental office, such as those with mobility issues or who live far away.

TYPES OF AT-HOME PROCEDURES THAT CAN BE DELIVERED SAFELY

Numerous types of procedures can be delivered safely through tele-dentistry when overseen by a licensed dental professional, including:

1. PROBLEM-FOCUSED CHECK-UPS AND CONSULTATIONS: These procedures can be conducted through video conferencing, allowing dental professionals to

diagnose and treat dental conditions remotely.

2. **FOLLOW-UP APPOINTMENTS:** Patients can have their treatment progress monitored remotely through tele-dentistry, reducing the need for in-person appointments.

3. **EMERGENCY CONSULTATIONS:** Tele-dentistry can be used to provide patients with urgent dental care advice and consultation when they are unable to physically visit a dental office.

4. **ORAL APPLIANCES:** Tele-dentistry has the unique ability to provide at-home dental services in the form of oral appliances such as night guards, clear aligners, remineralization trays, periodontal trays, and even tooth replacement through Valplast partial dentures.

It is very important to note, however, that these procedures are expected to be delivered at the SAME standard of care as the dental office. The dental professional needs to be licensed in the state where the patient is receiving care. The dental professional should also review the medical history, dental history, and other important data to determine the best course of treatment for the patient. This includes often requiring the patient to provide a copy of the latest radiographs and history of periodontal health for the patient.

REMOTE PATIENT MONITORING

Remote patient monitoring is another application of Tele-dentistry that has gained popularity in recent years. This approach involves the use of new technologies, such as mobile apps, sensors, and wearables, to provide constant data back to the dental professional.

This data can include information on a patient's brushing habits, gum health, and the use of dental appliances, among other things. Remote patient monitoring can help dental professionals monitor a patient's progress and provide timely interventions when necessary.

1. **REMOTE ORAL CANCER SCREENING:** Oral cancer screening is an essential aspect of dental care. Remote patient monitoring technology can enable dental professionals to conduct oral cancer screening remotely by leveraging images of the patient's mouth and teeth to identify any suspicious lesions or growths.

2. **REMOTE ORTHODONTIC MONITORING:** Orthodontic patients often require frequent check-ups to monitor the progress of their treatment. Remote patient monitoring technology can enable dental professionals to remotely monitor orthodontic patients' progress, reducing the need for in-person visits.

3. **REMOTE SLEEP APNEA MONITORING:** Sleep apnea is a common sleep disorder that can have serious oral health implications. Remote patient monitoring technology can enable dental professionals to remotely monitor patients with sleep apnea, providing data on their breathing patterns and identifying any issues that may require additional treatment.

4. **REMOTE PERIODONTAL DISEASE MONITORING:** Periodontal disease is a common oral health issue that can lead to tooth loss if left untreated. Remote patient monitoring technology can enable dental professionals to remotely monitor patients with periodontal disease, tracking the progression of the disease and adjusting treatment as necessary.

5. **REMOTE CAVITY DETECTION:** Early detection of cavities is critical to prevent the progression of decay. Remote patient monitoring technology can enable

dental professionals to remotely detect cavities by analyzing images of the patient's teeth and identifying areas of decay.

EMERGING TECHNOLOGIES

New technologies are transforming the tele-dentistry space, providing patients with access to more advanced dental services and tools. One example is the use of intraoral cameras, which can take high-quality images of a patient's mouth and teeth, allowing dental professionals to diagnose and treat dental conditions remotely.

Another example is the use of augmented reality, which can provide patients with a virtual simulation of their treatment outcome, helping them better understand their treatment options.

To ensure the effectiveness of tele-dentistry, dental professionals need access to high-quality equipment that can capture accurate images and videos of the patient's teeth and gums. From Artificial Intelligence to At-Home Intraoral Scanners, Tele-dentistry has transformed the field of dentistry, making it possible for patients to receive dental care from the comfort of their own homes. In addition to the Mouthcam at-home intraoral camera, several other hardware technologies have emerged that complement Tele-dentistry, including Artificial intelligence, smart mouth guards, and at-home intraoral scanners.

Artificial Intelligence (AI) has become a valuable tool in dentistry, providing dental professionals with more accurate diagnoses and treatment planning. AI can analyze data from x-rays, intraoral cameras, and other sources, providing dental professionals with valuable insights into the patient's oral health.

Artificial Intelligence can also help dental professionals identify potential issues before they become more serious, allowing for early intervention and prevention. Artificial Intelligence is particularly useful in tele-dentistry, where dental professionals need to rely on technology to provide accurate diagnoses and treatment plans remotely.

Smart mouth guards are another technology that complements tele-dentistry, providing dental professionals with a way to monitor a patient's oral health remotely. Smart mouth guards contain sensors that can measure the patient's bite force, temperature, and other factors that can indicate potential dental issues.

The data collected by the smart mouth guard can be transmitted to a dental professional, who can then provide advice and treatment remotely. Smart mouth guards are particularly useful for patients who are experiencing bruxism and sleep apnea.

At-home intraoral scanners are another technology that has emerged as a valuable complement to Tele-dentistry. These devices allow patients to take accurate 3D scans of their teeth and gums, which can be transmitted to a dental professional for review and diagnosis.

At-home intraoral scanners are particularly useful for patients who require orthodontic treatment, as the scans can be used to create custom aligners or other dental appliances. At-home intraoral scanners are also useful for patients who have difficulty traveling to a dental office or who live in remote or rural areas. These can come in the form of attachments to cell phones or the utilization of technology similar to intra-oral cameras such as the MouthCAM.

It is easy to see how and why Tele-dentistry is a rapidly growing field that is transforming the way dental care is delivered. It enables dental professionals to provide remote consultations, at-home dental exams, and other services, making dental care more accessible, affordable, and convenient for patients.

Tele-dentistry platforms like Dentulu leverage cutting-edge technologies, such as AI, augmented reality, and video conferencing, to provide patients with a personalized and interactive experience. Tele-dentistry can improve patient education by providing patients with more engaging and informative educational resources. It can also advance clinical collaboration between providers by enabling dental professionals to easily communicate and collaborate on patient care, regardless of their location.

Finally, the accessibility of Tele-dentistry is a significant advantage for patients in remote or rural areas who may have limited access to dental care. By improving access to care and reducing the overall cost of dental care, Tele-dentistry has the potential to improve oral health outcomes and expand access to care for patients around the world.

This is **LEADERSHIP volume 1, CHANGING THE WORLD FROM A DENTAL CHAIR** presented by ALPHA DENTISTRY. Welcome to the Alphas.

Dr. BAK NGUYEN

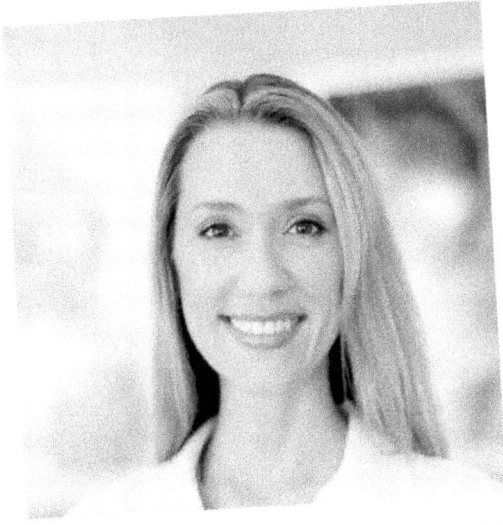

Dr. MARILYN SANDOR,
DDS, MS

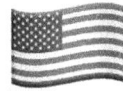

From the USA ■, **Dr. MARILYN SANDOR**, DDS, MS, is one of Southwest Florida's favourite paediatric dentists. She is highly experienced in her field, having founded her private practice, Naples Paediatric Dentistry in the beautiful community of Naples, Florida in 2001. Dr. Sandor is a successful business owner and an active member of her community. She is committed to educating her young patients on the importance of oral health and enjoys teaching children how to have healthy smiles for a lifetime. Dr. Sandor's paediatric-focused invention, Zooby prophy angles, inspired a full line of creative new products by Young Innovations which have been bringing joy to dental patients around the world for over a decade. She is the founder and CEO of GOODCHECKUP is the first Mobile to Mobile, Patent pending, Teledentistry solution that, gives dentists everywhere the ability to set themselves free from the standard care model and provide patients total convenience by placing access to care at their fingertips.

CHAPTER 19

"LEADERSHIP"

INSPIRE AND GET INSPIRED

By Dr. MARILYN SANDOR

When Dr. Bak Nguyen approached me to contribute a chapter in his upcoming book about leadership, I was truly humbled. When I asked if he was sure that he wanted to share this honour with me, I was deeply moved when Dr. Nguyen said that he invited me, because he saw me as a leader amongst our ranks and that he felt readers would be interested to hear about my journey and interesting events, such as why I had the opportunity to converse with the American Dental Association's Chief Economist about a solution I feel can change the way we address our dental health.

This encouragement reminded me that each of us has the potential to inspire another with our thoughts. Even if we are unaware of it, we may be inspiring someone else, who in turn inspires another, and by this chain reaction, we together move toward a new and better way.

My name is Marilyn Sandor, I am an experienced paediatric dentist and proud mother of three. I wake up happy and appreciate creativity. Now having been in practice for over two decades, I can say with certainty, that I am fortunate to have landed in a profession filled with pioneering spirits and imaginative innovators. I did not know how well it would suit me, until it did.

In elementary school, I would have a great deal of apprehension about getting called on to answer a question, but if the teacher asked us to share an idea, often I couldn't contain myself and would speak out of turn. That lack of self-control occasionally led to a scolding, but there were other times when my speaking out of turn would spur a discussion.

"Thought leadership is not about being the smartest person in the room. It's about having the courage to share your ideas and insights with others."

Dori Clarke

Because I believe that inspired ideas, inspire other great ideas, like a chain reaction, it is especially important to not let a potential spark of an idea get snuffed. Most of us have experienced a time where we held back from doing something we would like to do, out of fear of potential embarrassment. It's natural to feel insecure.

However, it can prevent us from taking risks and pursuing experiences that could be immensely rewarding. I have come to recognize that my own behaviour differs when it comes to topics about which I feel truly passionate. In those instances, my thoughts do not go to the negatives of why or why I should not. In these cases, I feel a sense of urgency to share. My natural instinct to help takes over.

"If I feel my solution has merit and it can solve a need, I become steadfast in presenting my ideas, even in the face of potential negative consequences."
Dr. Marilyn Sandor

While this can be challenging at times, I have found that it has allowed me to make a meaningful impact in areas that truly matter to me. I'll share a few examples of why speaking up, even when you might not be sure why you want to.

During my paediatric dental residency, I had the opportunity to pursue a Master's Degree, which required developing a thesis and presenting a Master's Thesis. At that time, it was customary for dental specialty program directors to recommend thesis topics, generally related to oral disease assessments.

However, I was drawn to a different area of study: the mindset of dental patients, particularly the mindset of the parents of children with extensive dental disease. I was curious as to why so few utilized preventive care and why our dental patients were almost resigned to seeking care only for emergency services.

I suggested that my thesis would investigate dental perceptions and how they affected the dental health of children. Keep in mind, this was nearly twenty-five years ago, and my program directors were not receptive to my idea. Despite the lack of support, I persisted, eventually finding a mentor, a psychologist in our dental college, and published my thesis, titled **"Relationship of Parents' Dental Indifference Level to Children's Oral Health."**

I am proud to say that my work inspired others, including my program directors, to publish more on the intersecting fields of paediatric dentistry and psychology, a relevant and important topic today. At the time I did not know the impact of this line of thinking; I just felt the drive to pursue it. I now see that I was right in my steadfastness and did contribute by leading others to further investigate this aspect of paediatric dentistry.

Upon finishing my residency, I decided that I had a different idea in mind for how a paediatric dental practice should feel than the outmoded, control-based style I experienced in our residency program. I wanted to help children feel that they were participants in the process of taking care of their own oral health and well-being; that it should bring them a sense of joy and hopefulness, because being healthy outweighs being unwell.

I opened my own practice in Southwest Florida, with lively, tropical colours. It looked and felt comfortable; with extra-soft dental chairs and with the office smelling nice, children were happy to watch movies on mounted televisions and enjoyed receiving prizes after every visit. It was my vision to make the user experience for each child fun and my outcomes were excellent.

About eight years into my practice ownership, I had an idea for a product that I felt would further engage my young patients' interest and acceptance of care. It turned out to be one of the first specifically for paediatric dentistry products for user experience.

It was not a paediatric-sized extraction forceps, nor was it a paediatric restraint, (which some of you may remember), rather it was a prophy angle designed to be cute. I made prototypes at my kitchen table and filed for a design patent. There was patience involved and a good deal of skepticism, however with the patent in hand, and a fair bit of insistence, an in-person visit with Young Innovations was arranged.

With a good presentation and awesome prototypes of the **Zooby Prophy Angles**, we were soon on the way. Inviting and fun for children, the prophy angles themselves look like zoo animal mascot characters. The prophy angles inspired not only a product line but a whole new division, which is paediatric-focused.

I am proud that people have been employed for nearly a dozen years because of my idea and that it has made visiting the dentist special for so many children around the world. This I feel is another example of why it is important to follow a gut feeling about a thought. It might end up leading an entire industry in a new direction!

This brings me to where this chapter started. What did I have to share with the American Dental Association's chief economist? To answer this, I will rewind to a few years back. Prior to the pandemic, my youngest child was diagnosed with type 1 diabetes. This condition requires the administration of insulin throughout the day, every day for her to live.

During the pandemic, there was a lot of alarming information in the news about "underlying conditions" and the increased risk for a negative outcome associated with them, which certainly scared me. There was plenty of fear to go around and many did not want to leave their homes. I was receiving phone calls and Facetime to give advice about dental concerns, which I was able to give, but it was of course not HIPAA compliant, and we did not have complete medical histories.

As a result, I decided to create something that would allow me to put my office in my hand. I decided that I wanted to create something to expand my reach and help other dentists everywhere also be able to offer advice and care to their patients.

I wanted to give us a tool to guide patients toward better oral health and be available in times of need. I imagined there would someday be home diagnostic kits, where all types of information could be shared virtually, in advance of a communication call. This became my new mission: to be part of leading dentistry into the digital age.

It was my intention to not stray far from the basic concept of tele-dentistry, which is the ability to connect a patient with a dentist for advice and care. From the patient's perspective, they can communicate with the dentist via their mobile phone. This was very important to me to achieve because mobile phones are ubiquitous.

From the standpoint of access and equity, it makes perfect sense. For dentists, tele-dentistry allows us to join the remote workforce and it has the potential to improve our dentist-patient relationship.

GoodCheckup was designed in a very specific way, at a very unique time, that no one never thought could happen. On the day I came home from the office, having been told to shut down, I immediately started thinking very deliberately about what I could possibly do. As a single mother of three who cares deeply about my dental practice and patients, but I was also truly scared, what was I supposed to do?

I thought to myself, what can I do without an office, without staff, without reliable internet to access patient records? Were there others like me?

> **"I have a brain, I have knowledge to share, a dentist is not just a manual labourer!"**
> Dr. Marilyn Sandor

I imagined the pediatricians, ready to go when equipped with a prescription pad in hand. All they need is a phone to call the pharmacy!

When I created **GoodCheckup** to be a stand-alone product for dentists who treat children, I meant it. Phone in hand only, a licensed paediatric dentist can provide advice and care, regardless of lockdowns or staff shortages. Regardless of geographical location or supply chain disruption, a secure communication tool, in my view, has value. Further, the fact that **GoodCheckup** would allow a paediatric dentist to be self-sufficient, sets them free!

Which brings us back to the beginning of this chapter, when I stated that I had the pleasure of speaking with Dr. Marko Vuijicic, the American Dental Association's Chief Economist. It is an honour to have spoken with him regarding his work and accomplishments. Dr. Vuijicic recently addressed the Senate and the discussion included the topic of tele-dentistry. I am thrilled to share that not only dentists and patients are eager to use technology to fill the voids in care distribution, but our own government has taken notice of the power technology can deliver to help its citizens have access to care.

I am proud to be on the cutting edge of this next progression in dentistry. It is my sincere hope that my stories have inspired you to reflect upon your own accomplishments and have given you more reason to share your ideas and bring them forward so that together we can reach great heights. In a nutshell, that is my definition of leadership. To inspire and find inspiration.

This is **LEADERSHIP volume 1, CHANGING THE WORLD FROM A DENTAL CHAIR** presented by ALPHA DENTISTRY. Welcome to the Alphas.

Dr. BAK NGUYEN

CHAPTER 20
"21ST CENTURY DENTISTRY"
WHAT GREAT TIMES WE ARE LIVING IN

By Dr. GURIEN DEMIRAQI

What great times we are living in! Technology is making it easier daily for us. I mean, one must be amazed by what one can do with a simple smartphone and the latest PC. Our work has changed, starting from the apps for appointments and how to handle the numerous equipment needs and finances easily. Lately, even the front desk is simplified with Artificial Intelligence secretaries or online handling remotely. Explaining the procedures to patients with interactive videos and animations make it so much easier to help them understand and get accepted the treatment plan.

You can take pictures to give the patient an idea of what he or she will get at the end of the treatment in real-time, including smile design and soft tissues, is such a blessing, to both parties. Accurate colour-matched with several devices, 3D printers to print and create any type of lab prosthetics, all of those made dentistry more interesting and surely more convenient.

In orthodontics, treatments like Invisalign make it predictable and more accurate to change patient smiles on a daily basis. Not to forget about how the most difficult parts: implantology planning and prosthetic are facilitated with the various programs and technologies evolving on a daily basis. Sometimes, I wonder how did we succeed before!?

Back in the day, I needed half a day to preprogram surgery and implants. Now, it is done in less than half an hour. Before, you needed to take impressions, have a lab to make models, and only then, you could plan the surgery. Nowadays, I take impressions with digital scanners, and match the CBCT imaging to it, in a matter of minutes. Doing so, I can plan with even more accuracy and from there, have a better overall prediction, implant placement possibilities etc. I have to add that this technology is getting more and more accurate daily.

For some years now, robots like Yomi and similar are placing implants, almost without the need for human intervention and with great accuracy. Even mentoring is becoming much easier nowadays. In complex surgeries, with the help of cameras in the dental units and zoom-like connections, it is now possible to receive help in real-time from mentors during surgery, even if there are from another continent. This is how far we have gone.

The dental units are compressing more and more information in such a small space and are becoming more and more interactive and capable of assisting dentists in their daily functions.

One can argue that it all costs money. I agree, but I will state that competition is strong and the prices are going down and will go down even more in the near future. One key advantage is the time-saving these technologies allow. Many procedures are getting automated, most of the procedures are now done in office, without the need to send the patient anywhere else. Which is the best way to keep the patient happy and in-house.

All this tech, of course, will come with the cost of losing jobs, the need for training and knowledge in fields that traditional dentists know little or nothing about. On the plus side, this will simplify and standardize many procedures, that nowadays are done only by elite dentists and top dental laboratories with high costs of planning and production. Who can stand in the way of evolution and progress?

Let me clarify. We need to evolve! Dentistry was seen for a long time as a "lone Ranger" kind of job. Meaning that a dentist is being very good and performs everything, from hygiene to complex and difficult surgeries, prosthetics and orthodontics with ease and excellence.

Well, we all know that this is only a utopia. The trouble starts with that lie since no one (and I mean no one) can be good at all of these tasks! One can be good at some of them and not so good at others. That's okay, that's reality.

That brought the need for specializations which made one more capable in one or several branches of dentistry. This model has worked well in the USA and still, is finding footing in Europe and in Asia. With the advent of technology coming to the rescue, dentists are mistakenly thinking that AI and technology will make it possible to be a super dentist and do everything right! Nothing can be further from the truth!

Those technologies will help reduce time, improve efficiency and even achieve some tasks, until now, out of reach. But this all comes with a cost! When Henry Ford automatized the automobile industry, it helped tremendously, but this happened because there was a big demand for the product. In this case, the demand for cars was great and conventional production couldn't meet with demand. His automatization process was welcomed because it solved a big problem.

Applying the same logic, do we need dental products to be produced more rapidly? Is there a demand for that? And what problem are we solving? If you handle for 8 patients a day in a single dentist's office, why would you need an oral scanner that can scan in 2 minutes but increase the financial overhead of your clinic while taking an impression the traditional way takes 10 minutes and won't add hundred and thousands of expenses on your monthly ledger?

The oral scanner needs a variety of new tech to complement and finish the required task (all of which cost even more money). All of that in the name of saving time! What will do with that time saved?

"It all comes down to money!"
Murray Walker

This means essentially: do we have enough patients to accommodate and use the new tech? My answer: alone you don't! So, what should we do? Do the hard thing, what we turn a blind eye to: we have to let our Ego go and to unite.

We all have an Ego. Sometimes, it is so big that it takes over the best of us, blinding us for what would be best for us! Ego, that's the only reason that we deny the obvious. Together we are better, we complement one another in more than 1 way. But we are already doing that, will you say! Sure, we go to meetings, events and international congresses, we talk about cases and problems we solved or didn't solve. But still, we are very resilient and struggle to work together within the same structure. Everyone wants to be a *Prima donna*, not to follow "orders" from a colleague, even when deep down, we know they are right.

"The lone ranger mentality from the 19th century does not work in the 21st century!"

Dr. Gurien Demiraqi

Only by uniting can we divide the operational costs, increase productivity and have enough demand to justify the purchase of better technology. Uniting is a win-win situation. The sooner we realize that and adapt, the better.

Otherwise, with the fast advancement in technology, some if not many of us will be left behind wondering… what if! The truth is that patients want better, faster and cheaper care. And as soon as those are available, they will jump ship. We can either adapt and facilitate the trend or stay behind with our old ship rusting. Learn from the newspapers and magazine giants that once ruled the world!

The near future belongs to larger organizations, composed of several capable professionals able to handle all the tasks and challenges in a timely fashion.

To meet these kinds of standards, one has to operate within a team. To adapt to newer technology and to gain more financial weight (cutting on our liabilities) we need to unite. All those who will not adapt to this reality will slowly disappear.

This is **LEADERSHIP volume 1, CHANGING THE WORLD FROM A DENTAL CHAIR** presented by ALPHA DENTISTRY. Welcome to the Alphas.

Dr. BAK NGUYEN

CHAPTER 21
"TAKING CONTROL"
DENTAL COMPANIES CAN HELP THEMSELVES AND THE WHOLE INDUSTRY
By Dr. MAHSA KHAGHANI

To learn from the great experts the latest techniques as well as the most advanced technologies, and to apply them in our daily practice is the key to evolution. On that matter, I believe that dental companies are key players. In my opinion, dental companies should be much more involved in dental training rather than spending millions on marketing.

"Education will sell itself!"
Dr. Mahsa Khaghani

If all of them dedicate an important part of the investment they make annually in marketing into training dentists, their means will spread as much, if not even at a faster rate while diminishing their risk/exposure ratio. In fact, the simple and direct extension to learning is applying. In other words, to implement that new technology and standard of care.

Since dentists all around the world have mandatory hours to spend in continuous education, making them accessible and affordable is a sure way to win the heart of the profession. I know, they are already doing that, but I believe that they could do so much more!

After 12 years of my life dedicated to training post-graduate doctors, I can affirm for a fact that investment in formation is directly leading to the sale of that product, if proven effective. And the relationship is mutually beneficial, for private companies, doctors, and ultimately, the patients. Earlier, I mentioned the standard of care. Well, the more a product or a technique is used, the faster it becomes a standard of care. Isn't that the dream and goal of each private company, to be the standard in the market? As Dr. Bak said, to price below the resistance point, if companies are making their training and products below the resistance point, it should be a win-win for everyone.

With this, I want to call on all dental companies to stop and analyze the expense that they are devoting to high-level training. If all companies had qualified dentists in their company dedicated to the analysis and selection of the best experts related to the products they offer, they would see that the investment they make in them would be the one that would offer them the best return.

Actually, this goes well beyond selling. Dental companies also have a very important role in the creation of experts and leaders in dentistry. For a dentist to be able to dedicate himself or herself to quality training and show doctors their follow-up with extensive documentation and case study is the most convincing way to educate and prove a point.

With that in mind, what company can afford for the market to eventually share their results and organize themselves to teach what they just mastered? That is such a long and ineffective process! If dental companies are taking the lead in recruiting their experts, subsidizing them for training, documentation and, eventually, teaching, they will have taken upon the most beneficial bet on their ledger.

Dentists may have the best training, but in order to develop and share their experience in lectures, they will need significant support in advance regarding the cost of the products in use. For this reason, I also consider it important that all companies have an annual budget dedicated to doctors who are going to develop their products in clinics and who can become KOL (Key Opinion Leader) of their brand.

"The creation of leaders in our profession is essential for our daily progress."

Dr. Mahsa Khaghani

But these leaders must have excellent prior training and for this, having access to products for the application on their patients is crucial. Documenting cases is essential so that later they can train more colleagues.

The leaders that we have in Dentistry in each specialty, must have continuous support from the companies with which they collaborate so that they can increasingly offer higher quality courses and be able to spread their knowledge worldwide.

Once dental companies have opinion leaders using their products, they must keep good care of them as assets, continuously evolving and improving their techniques and clinical results. That is common and good practice to maintain and increase their sale and market shares.

With all that said, I believe that dentistry and its development would not be feasible if we did not have large dental companies that make an important and continuous effort to be able to offer us better products and more advanced technologies every day. But in order to move forward, the relationship should be strengthened, at least tenfold. Especially now that the dental industry is at the crossroads of evolution.

This is **LEADERSHIP volume 1, CHANGING THE WORLD FROM A DENTAL CHAIR** presented by ALPHA DENTISTRY. Welcome to the Alphas.

Dr. BAK NGUYEN

CHAPTER 22

"K.O.L. NEEDED"

LEADERSHIP LIES IN EXPERIENCE

By Dr. MAHSA KHAGHANI

In order to move forward, we need leaders. But what is a leader nowadays? What is a K.O.L. in the dental field? The figure of opinion leaders in our profession is really important to help and motivate us to be better professionals every day. Our job, after all, is one that often involves spending many hours alone in our clinic with our patients and we get used to a series of rituals in each procedure we perform.

Just like the rest of the population, many dentists are very resistant when it comes to change their routines and habits. But wait a minute, how can you do better if you refuse to change what you are doing now? That's the biggest mistake we are trapped in: to have protocols acting as barriers to prevent improvement in our practice! I know, it sounds contra-productive and yet, this is our reality, to every single one of us.

After so many years working as a dentist and being lucky enough to meet with so many dentists from all around the world, I have unfortunately realized that change is a very difficult topic to address.

"Everyone agrees with doing better, but no one is ready to change what they currently do!"

Dr. Mahsa Khaghani

And the excuse? Well, if it isn't broken, why fix it? That's the common theme! Well, it doesn't have to be broken to slow you down or to be inefficient! And here is where a K.O.L. is making a difference in your life.

A K.O.L. is also a practitioner, just like you. He or she knows the actual protocol and made it better by implementing this or that. Just like you, they need concrete proof of the improvement and are basically sharing those with you in their seminar. It is more about sharing than about teaching! Now, you just have the testimony and the documentation of someone who used to do exactly what you are doing right now, of someone who understands the pain and the frustration of what you are enduring right now! With a K.O.L., it is not about change but about solving your frustrations and limitations. Do I really have to say more?

That is also why, there is practically no selling needed, almost no resistance. It's all about implanting a solution or, in other words, solving a frustration of yours! Now, more than ever, we need more passionate masters, K.O.L. to inspire and motivate dentists to look beyond their habits and what they have accepted as a necessary evil! It doesn't have to be that way, there is better! From my perspective, that should raise the standard of care and renew your passion as a practitioner. It did for me!

As a director of post-graduate programs in dentistry, both in Madrid and in New York, I can't stretch enough the importance of great continuous training. It is the only way to improve the quality of dentistry, aka the standard of care. Quality continuing education should be mandatory for all dentists, but the high cost is often an obstacle for many of them. And that's the opportunity I am presenting to all the major dental companies out there!

WHO CAN BECOME A LEADER IN DENTISTRY?

To become a leader in our profession, dentistry, is much easier than one might think. But the first question I would ask you would be, what is a leader for you?

It is very important that a person who dedicates himself or herself to this profession constantly wants to be a better professional and to offer the best of him or herself. In simple words, you need passion. Unfortunately, some of us have faded their passion along the way. And again, that is why they should invest in great training programs with K.O.L. infused with passion! That should kickstart the renewal of their passion and commitment to the profession.

The first thing you should do as a dentist is to see if you like the discipline you are doing, even if it inspires you to push further. If that isn't the case, my recommendation is that you try to access training where you can learn enough notions from the other disciplines of dentistry and find one that suits you better. Be honest with yourself. More than once, I saw people after years of practice and a specialty degree, find their passion by switching to another branch of dentistry. Well, if that keeps you happy and motivated, why wait or hesitate?

Actually, the worst thing that can happen is for one to stay stuck in a position, unfulfilled and unhappy. To go to the office and to look at the clock, looking to "punch out" is the worst that can happen to any of us.

There are many hours that we dedicate to our profession which require much precision for optimal results. We do not have the right to make mistakes. Add to that that you have to be confident for your patient and your team while performing at the best of your abilities, all of which take much energy. We treat people, remember? They feel what we feel. And if you are unhappy sitting there, it is a bad start! Connecting with a passionate K.O.L. will break that bad circle!

Sure, a great environment will help, but the most important part is how we feel and see ourselves. That will reflect immediately on the people we are providing care to. To find ways to keep you motivated to come in the office every morning, to greet your team and your patients as important guests, as friends, to find the time and the passion to improve your environment, just to make it more pleasant, a little more efficient, a little more pretty, that translates into making everyone's life better. Well, you are a leader!

In my experience, it is important that you set clear and well-defined objectives to implement, that will help monitor the progress and keep you happy along the way. It might seem like a stretch, but believe me, once you reach that kind of satisfaction in your career, that energy transposes to other aspects of your life too!

"To become a leader, as a dentist, is a goal that every doctor should have. You do that to find your happiness."
Dr. Mahsa Khaghani

Then, we need you to inspire others to do the same, to set themselves free from the depression and to renew their passion for our profession. That is for the good of our patience, the good of our profession and our own happiness!

Sure, that will not come in one day. No one is born a leader. In our field, we need to earn our stripes. Being a great master and reference in Dentistry is not an easy job.

As I mentioned before, obviously it first requires a first phase where you must train thoroughly, then have the possibility of applying all the notions you have acquired by documenting clinical cases through which you will then be able to share within seminars and classrooms. This can be easier with the support of the medical companies involved.

With your own experience seeing better patients outcome, passion and magic will fill your heart and you will be happy. To increase that happiness, share it by teaching it to your peers! Guess what? You are even happier! Then, as you feel happy and fulfilled, you will be asking for more!

Even for those with a fear of speaking in public, you are a doctor, so you have no problem talking to a small crowd of people. Start there, and as you grow, you will be addressing a whole auditorium before you notice! Once you feel happy and fulfilled, nothing is out of reach. Focus on your happiness and what you are good at!

"The key is passion!"

Dr. Mahsa Khaghani

The last point that I would like to highlight is that in addition to the training and the way in which the doctor is going to transmit his knowledge, it is important that he has advice on how to make his presentations and how to teach his knowledge in an attractive and modern way.

What happens many times is that we have great world experts who unfortunately are not able to sell out their programs because they are not able to prepare presentations that are attractive enough so that the attendees stay alert during the lecture and many times that translates to unattractive courses, despite the fact that the content is excellent.

I always recommend hiring experts, coaches and designers to learn and master their craft. No one is good everywhere. What is important is to get the needed help to be able to share the greatness we hold inside. Don't assume that it is not important, don't underestimate anything. By the end of the day, your role was to make your patient happy, you did that. That also made you happy.

Now, your goal is to get your peers to share your enthusiasm and happiness. If you need some help to polish your speaking skills, that's a very good deal! Remember, by the end of it, you will be the one coming out the happiest!

I am sorry, but I have to say it, there is a lot of EGO in our profession. There are also so many dentists who, professionally speaking, could be better, at developing in different aspects. And they are not happy. What is pinning them down is often, if not almost, their EGO. During all my years in the profession, the wisest people I met were precisely those who share that you can never say that you know enough about something.

"There is always a way to get better. Hey, that's hope! That's youth! That's happiness!"

Dr. Mahsa Khaghani

In the name of hope, of happiness, for the sake of our profession, drop the EGO! You will thank me one day.

This is **LEADERSHIP volume 1, CHANGING THE WORLD FROM A DENTAL CHAIR** presented by ALPHA DENTISTRY. Welcome to the Alphas.

Dr. BAK NGUYEN

CHAPTER 23
"MILLION DOLLAR MINDSET"
KEY OPINION LEADERS

By Dr. BAK NGUYEN

Until now, we've been dwelling much into the problems of our profession. How about bringing in some hope? Before being known as an Alpha, I was known for my **MILLION DOLLAR MINDSET** series. That is both a series of books and Podcasts. Actually, that Podcast series is my most popular brand, addressing ways to help entrepreneurs and leaders to grow.

How about bridging the mindset of Alphas with the MILLION DOLLAR? Until now, we've been busy trying to cure and rebuild our profession, of caring for the world. Would it be okay to do that while moving forward with financial success at the same time? Actually, that is the key ingredient of **MILLION DOLLAR MINDSET**: to bridge the need of the many with concrete solutions.

So how do we do that, addressing dentistry? Let's go back to Dr. Khaghani's vision of having Key Opinion Leaders (K.O.L.) to further the advancement of our profession with the sponsorship of dental companies. This is a great idea, but someone still needs to convince these companies of the return on investment of sponsoring K.O.L.

How about proving to these big companies that this is the way to win big? Bear with me. As a host, I am fortunate to constantly meet with new people. As an entrepreneur, I am very fortunate to constantly meet with great people. When you add the 2 together, I have the opportunity to meet, learn from, and connect with great leaders and innovators.

Last year, I had the privilege to meet Frank Baylis, a successful entrepreneur and business leader, known for his innovative approach to business strategy and his commitment to corporate responsibility. As president of Baylis Medical Company, he has built a reputation for driving growth and success through a combination of strategic vision, operational excellence, and customer focus.

Born and raised in Montreal, Frank Baylis began his career in the family business, founded by his mother. The company started as an importer of medical devices. Over the years, it grew into a designer and manufacturer of medical devices that are sold around the world. Under Frank's leadership, the company quickly changed from distributor to innovator.

In 1999, Frank joined Baylis Medical Company, a company that specialized in the design and production of innovative products for the healthcare industry. As Vice President of Sales and Marketing, he played a key role in the company's growth, helping to build a strong customer base and expand into new markets.

In 2001, Frank was promoted to President and he immediately set about transforming the company's operations and culture. He led a successful rebranding effort, launched several new product lines, and implemented lean manufacturing processes that improved efficiency and profitability. Under his leadership, Baylis Medical Company became a recognized leader in the healthcare industry, known for its high-quality products and customer-centric approach.

With Frank's vision, the company expanded its product portfolio, diversified its customer base, and led a major international expansion effort. At the same time, he has remained committed to Baylis Medical Company's core values of corporate responsibility, environmental sustainability, and ethical business practices.

In 2022, he sold a division of Baylis Industries for 1.75 Billion US Dollars. He made that, designing and creating new medical devices. That's 23 years after he joined the company and 17 years after he re-oriented his company from distribution to designing. Well, 17 years is a long time most will say. But not in the medical field, especially when you are trying to introduce new designs and concepts.

My exact question to Frank was: "H̦ow did you manage to advance so quickly in a field so filled with red tapes, as conservative as the surgical field?" Well, he smiled and gave me 3 letters as an answer: K.O.L.

What you should know about Frank Baylis, is that he is a true leader. He was elected as a member of the Parliament of Canada a few years ago. In his career, he sold many divisions of Baylis Industries, the 1.75 billion was only his last success, making him the latest Canadian Billionaire (by the end of 2022). So it wasn't, 3 letters that made the success of M. Baylis. K.O.L., these letters were the key to his rise. For decades, Frank always had a suitcase ready in his office, for emergencies, in the advent that he received a call from a surgeon somewhere in North America, sometimes, even from further. Then, the surgeons call and he will be flying in, with a moment's notice, to assist the "experimental surgery". He will provide as much support as possible, but as he put it himself, he is an engineer, not a doctor.

Well, because he supported the surgeons, the operations made breakthroughs and history. The surgeons gave keynotes and speaking events, bragging about their merits.

These inspired other doctors to call Frank to apply his devices in other medical situations. They too, made breakthroughs and history. And they too, went on to brag about their pioneering work, all with the help of Baylis Industries's devices and Frank by their side. They were leaders who became K.O.L. (Key Opinion Leaders). They were his most trusted ambassadors.

And that success story made Frank Baylis into a Billionaire. Sure the money is impressive, but what is even more, is how Frank achieved such level of success, with a suitcase waiting in his office, even as president. Today, Frank keeps the same approach, he stays humble and is always ready to jump in and help. This really is a **MILLION DOLLAR MINDSET**. And he was kind enough to share it with me.

"K.O.L., that's the answer you are looking for."

Frank Baylis

This completely changed my approach to addressing the reforms that our industry deeply needs. I was already empowering international collaborations. Now, armed with the K.O.L. power, thanks to M. Baylis, I am doubling down on this culture of empowering and of sharing, which are the keys to the ALPHAS. Gratitude Frank. I hope you will be proud of what you've inspired.

CEOs, Presidents, Vice-Presidents, and Board Members, save on your marketing budget and trade shows deployments, find and nurture your next K.O.L. and support them as they operate. Empower them to share their success with their colleagues in conferences and keynotes. Professor Nagy and Dr. Khaghani hold the key to so many of them in Europe and in North America for such WIN-WIN-WIN situations.

This is **LEADERSHIP volume 1, CHANGING THE WORLD FROM A DENTAL CHAIR** presented by ALPHA DENTISTRY. Welcome to the Alphas.

Dr. BAK NGUYEN

CHAPTER 24
"HUMANIZING DENTISTRY"
BEYOND TEETH AND GUMS
By Dr. BAK NGUYEN

Now on to another facet of leadership in dentistry. Sure it is cool and glamorous to speak about leadership and **MILLION DOLLAR MINDSET**. Writing the first book of **CHANGING THE WORLD FROM A DENTAL CHAIR**, back in 2018, I had a much different concern in mind: the depression rate within our ranks.

Prior to that book, I addressed the issue within my 5th opus: **PROFESSION HEALTH, THE UNCONVENTIONAL QUEST TO HAPPINESS**, co-written with Dr. Mirjana Sindolic and Dr. Robert Durand. I invite you to look those up. To summarize the theme, I was dwelling on why we, dentists, are so prompted to depression and suicide. That is not me speaking, but the statistics within our ranks for the last few decades. It is so that we still greet the new dental students with that anecdote. Well, that's how I was greeted in the profession, more than 25 years ago.

I tried to address the issue. Looking in the mirror, I saw no depression no desire for worse looking back at me. Me, a sensitive soul who became a doctor to honour the wish of his immigrant parents? Me, who came to rise as an anchor and a world top 100 doctor by 2021? How did I survive all of this? How did I thrive as a dentist?

What I can tell you is that I gain the favour of the financial industries looking to empower and heal my peers and colleague. Sadly, my peers did not respond much to the quest of happiness. Instead, they responded pretty strongly as I laid on the MILLION DOLLAR theme. With that, I got their attention. This was prior to COVID, prior to the creation of the ALPHAS.

That shocked me, even hurt me. Are money and financial success that important to us, dentists, above our mental health and life? After years of researching why are dentists so prompt to depression and suicide, I finally found the answer, while researching in another industry. I will refrain from sharing that answer and logic in here, since it would be the topic of a following book with Professor Bennete Fernandes of Malaysia, and Professor Sandra Fabiano, of Brazil. I apologize for the suspense.

What I will share with you though is that I avoid much of the depression of our profession because I was deeply invested in connecting with my patients. What I did from instincts and for my own survival, I developed into philosophy:

"I treat people, not teeth."

Dr. Bak Nguyen

That mentally pushed me to evolve and to adapt it to my international collaboration with the ALPHAS. Writing the **ALPHA DENTISTRY** series, having 10-12 international Key Opinion Leaders to answer the same list of frequently asked questions (FAQ), I realized that I was doing just that, humanizing our profession.

My goal was to create the first dental crowd-sourcing knowledge base to help democratize our field. What I realized, is that FAQ is the best way to humanize our science into skills, human skills. Professor Nagy stated that fact with such clarity: we are not trained for communication. Even if she tried to address that as a professor and a dean, the students' interest was more toward surgical skills.

Well, any experienced doctor will tell you that empathy and communication are top clinical skills to master on the ground. This is also why it was so easy to write that FAQ series with experienced practitioners. The key here is experience.

Linking the dots together, I realized that answering patients' questions was one of my main functions as a doctor. Taking the time to have them follow the logic and understand made me the loved and successful doctor that I am today. And the more I am loved, the happier I am, and the further I am from depression. Does that start to make any sense to you too?

FAQ answering is the exercise of putting science into words that the patients will understand. Even better, the logic was triggered by them. Give them satisfaction and you will have gained a new friend! Following that line of thought, I started wondering if we were not on the verge of a remedy to help the future generation of dentists and their patients.

What if, together, we develop a new norm to have our new graduates shaped and trained in how to face their patients, having them to answer FAQ? That will provide them with the ultimate test before being on their own, facing a concerned or scared patient!

Sure, we all learnt that with the years, and still, our depression rates are through the roof. What if, from the beginning of our dental career, we started gathering the love and respect of our patients, won't that set all of our members in the right direction?

Will that be a new certification, a new exam, or a course to be added to the curriculum? This has to be discussed amongst the Alpha visionaries within the next years. But the idea stands: let's better prepare our new members to be loved and welcomed by society at large!

That last part, well, COVID proved to all of us how far we are from general trust and love... Humanizing dentistry is a noble goal. After the latest crisis, it is now a must. The norm of FAQ is a means to an end. Well, a pretty cool one if you ask me.

What are your thoughts? To make this one work, we will need all the help we can gather. Within the Alphas alone, we are so many deans and experienced teachers. We do have the influence to save lives. This time, it will be the lives within our ranks!

This is **LEADERSHIP volume 1, CHANGING THE WORLD FROM A DENTAL CHAIR** presented by ALPHA DENTISTRY. Welcome to the Alphas.

Dr. BAK NGUYEN

CHAPTER 25
"OPTIMIZING DENTISTRY"
LET'S CUT THE FAT AND THE WASTE
By Dr. BAK NGUYEN

With a century of advancement in technology, we should have seen a decrease in dental fees, to follow common logic and Dr. Demiraqi's observation. That makes sense on paper. In reality, the advent of new technologies has only contributed to increasing the operational costs of dentists throughout the world. Dentistry today, has never been that expensive!

And why is that? Well, Dr. Demiraqi summarized it into one single word: EGO. We all have egos. Some a bigger than others, but our egos have been our biggest flaws. Then, the industries built on that, selling to those of us their best technology, empowering those with better technology to be the king of the hill, for a short instant. Then, they go to our neighbours and colleagues and empower them to catch up, not to be left behind... until the next technological invention.

These machines are expensive. If they allow more precision and great time saving, who is benefiting from that? A very narrow portion of the patients of that doctor, not even all of his or her patients. That's for the precision advancement. About the time-saving? Well, it gets rapidly lost once the team in place gets tired and pauses for the rest of the week…

So in theory, science and technology made dentistry better. That's true! Why have they contributed to increase the honorarium instead of decreasing it as planned? Well, because of ego leading to individualism leading to tremendous waste. This is the ugly portrait of our industry. Because of that general trend in the industry, the waste of each dental clinic is averaged by the national board that then, recommends the reasonable honorarium as national guidelines… and now, it has become an acceptable norm!

This does not make any sense! How would you feel if each physician needs his or her own MRI machine? What would you think of each physician owning their own operation room? Well, we, as dentists, have deployed 3 clinics at each corner street (figure of speech… but not too far from reality) in which, we own 3 or more operation rooms, which are empty more than 50% of the time since we can only work for as much… and then, post-covid, we faced staff shortage…

Wait, that's not all! We do own our x-ray machine and sensors, our digital and CBCT machine and what else have we bought in the name of medicine, in the name of our patients, but really to feed our ego?

Sharing, that's the word you are looking for. That's the word we do not know within our ranks. To fix our industry and leverage technology to lower at large our honorarium, we need to change our mindset and ways to deploy our resources on the field. The only way to cut the fees to patients is to cut our operational costs first! Reduction in salary? That would be suicidal and the worse alternative possible. So since salary is only going up and we are a service industry, heavily dependant on staff, what do we do?

How about grouping together for purchase power and to cut down on waste? My company, Mdex & Co. was created on these principles. We package the best and most comfortable hotel for dentists to allow them to be at their best, giving them ownership, while cutting down on their cost of production (waste).

For those of you interested, my 7th book, **CHANGING THE WORLD FROM A DENTAL CHAIR** was written to defend my nomination as Ernst and Young Entrepreneur of the Year 2018. I ended up losing that one, but the ideas went out to gain the hearts and attention of the financial world. Then, COVID hit. But that is another story…

Back to our deployment issues, we all want to be the boss. That's fine, it can be arranged. We all want to be independent, our licensing bureaus are pushing for it. That too can be arranged. We have great credit scores and the means to build (on that, trust me, spend some time with me and all banks will see your value). What we lack is the financial intelligence and the humility to make sense of our numbers.

Financially speaking, everything that you are buying is losing value as soon as it is installed, just like a new car. The more expensive, the steeper the fall. Even your clinics, your installations, walls and light fixture, everything is losing in value. Unless you bought the building in which you operate, the highest value you had was when you bought it!

Now, what is gaining in value is your team and your growing clientele. Well, can you sell your team? Can you sell your patients? It does not even sound right to raise the question! In business terms, the business people found ways to package those into ratios and value. That goes for your clientele. They called it buying and transferring goodwill. On the staff, nothing can really be packaged.

That's better than nothing will you say! Wait a minute, the goodwill that you are building, well, those are based on you! On your services and the trust people have in you! Once you leave, that goodwill melts faster than ice under the sun! Is that a good investment? Bankers and investors will qualify those as risky. What is safe is to bet on every single doctor!

In other words, you are the asset! You, are the business! That is the financial wisdom that was never taught to anyone of us. We were empowered and told to build, buying liabilities and piling them up. Since we have access to credit, we buy and sit on depreciating assets, only to look better than our peers next door. As soon as we finished paying for a piece of equipment (which we utilize less than 50% of the time while paying for it 100% plus interest), our accountants are advising us to buy something else for the fiscal expenses column on our tax report. And, there is always a new piece of technology available on the market...

And that is the rat race for which we are signing up. This has nothing to do with patient care, passionate dentistry, and the reason why, in the first place, we became doctors. Our intentions were good, but the current state of the industry and its trends corrupted each and every one of us. In turn, that financial burden is transferred in the increase of honorarium, we are vassal states to our banks, and we live with the lie of being a business owner! You own liabilities and you are the business! By the way, we are not even good business managers... because we are doctors!

You don't believe me? Please, take an hour or 2, just to research and study the statistics of our profession. From the general perception of the population to our rate and prominence to depression and suicide!

And that spiral has evolved freely in our industry of Dental Medicine, for now, more than a century. The public demands changes. If the change is not coming from within, well, it will be coming from outsiders.

The best example that I can quote is the transformation of orthodontic expertise. From the advent of invisalign which utilizes computers and state-of-the-art manufacturing processes to democratize orthodontics amongst dentists, within a decade, the trend gave birth to a cheaper alternative without dentists!

"If you think that our licences and exclusive rights will protect us, think again!"

Dr. Bak Nguyen

Covid shows us how insignificant we are to the rest of medicine and what the general public thinks of us. Well, since Covid and the shortage of staff that followed, did you know that governments are the ones pushing for artificial intelligence and automatization of all industries, across the board? They are not only pushing for it, they are financing it!

In such a context, how much longer will we stay attached to our ego and old ways, hoping that things will be back to normal. And even then, at what normality are you referring to? Our rat race and depression rate?

This has to end here and now. And the first thing to do is to stop our denials. Then, we need to listen to our patients and see what is important to them. We think that our clinic and installation are the most precious. Ask them and listen actively to their answers. They value you and what you can do for them! Everything else is accessories and depreciating in value.

Then, sit down with your financial adviser and ask them to tell you your worth in financial terms. Listen to his or her answers, but above all, listen to the logic. Instead of being offended, see the trend and how the rest of the world is looking at us, at least from a financial standpoint.

Then, ask yourself if your EGO was worth all of the burden and sacrifices. If you come to the same conclusion as I did, well, let's start a dialogue. We can start rebuilding.

This is **LEADERSHIP volume 1, CHANGING THE WORLD FROM A DENTAL CHAIR** presented by ALPHA DENTISTRY. Welcome to the Alphas.

Dr. BAK NGUYEN

CHAPTER 26

"THE WIND OF CHANGE"

WHAT AWAITS AHEAD

By Dr. BAK NGUYEN

No one can stand against progress for long and think that they can win, just like no one can stand against nature. Empires rose and fell from shifts in technology. The Roman Empire had engineering and roads until these same roads led the enemies to the heart of Rome to be ravaged, again and again. The British Empire had her ships, until armies grew wings with aviation.

Who are we, dentists, to think that we are above the wind of change? We embraced the Industrial Age by reforming our dental schools and support systems (dental companies). As dentists, we learnt to delegate allowing hygienists and denturists to join our profession. But that is all we learnt from the Industrial Age, we remained artisans when it comes to the practice of our science.

The Information Age passed us by. Sure, we now have websites and screens in all of our operatories, but we are still holding tight to information as if it was state secret. Well, we can be blamed here, since personal medical information is state secret. But we, as dentists, applied that secrecy to all of our information stocked on private encrypted servers. We did not learn anything from the Information Age, only to burden ourselves with more liabilities and norms to comply with.

If some fields in dentistry are doing better than others nowadays, orthodontics and implantology are amongst leaders. And why is that so? Because these 2 have been upgraded by outsiders and propelled our means deep into the Information Age!

These are not just fancy words, but the true evolution and shift operating under our feet as we debate. With robotics in implantology and direct-to-customer orthodontic appliances, we are not the ones defining dental medicine, we are defined by its advancement.

The lawmakers and licensing bureaus won't be the ones defining what will come next either, they will only react to implanted changes. If you need a clear proof of that, follow the news about artificial intelligence in the Spring of 2023. That brings me to the conclusion that change will not happen because we need it. Change will not happen because decided so. Change comes because it was made possible and people made the choice to consume the easier, cheaper, smarter, and perhaps, even stronger, alternatives. And the People are always right!

In concise terms, the change needed for us to rebuild our profession will not come from our leadership or licensing bureaus. It can come from our education system, but that will take a radical change in mentality. The most probable source of change will come from the advancement in technology. These advancements in technology were all made by outsiders of our industry.

Well, this time, I propose that we are part of the leadership of change. That we embrace openness and surf the waves to implement the technology that will serve our patients and decrease the financial burden for both parties. I proposed that we extend our hand to outside expertise and build with them the bridges to the future.

The alternative is to leave all of that power and influence to define the future of our profession to complete strangers. Don't get me wrong, the outsiders are not the enemies. Before making it into our field, all they wanted was to collaborate with us to better customize their products and services. That is financial wisdom since it diminishes their risks.

Well, in the past, we stayed on our high horses, looking down on them. Then, they decided to move forward without us, leaving it to the general public and the laws in commerce to pick a winner and a loser. Is this all that we are? Guardian of old ways waiting to the wear down by evolution and the same public we swore to protect?

On that, allow me to raise a hard question: are we protecting the public as we are ignoring the progress and future possibilities?

As for my part, I am directing the Alpha Dentistry series of books in that manner: to gather the first crowdsourcing wisdom of our profession. That also means leaving secrecy behind and embracing the democratization of our science, amongst us and with the general public.

This will be a first within our ranks. That series of books is the most ambitious and inclusive project ever attempted in the history of dentistry. If you think that this is advancement, well, think again. It is merely playing catch-up! Wikipedia was built on that model for all of the human knowledge more than a quarter of a century ago! We are not as smart as we like to think.

With data in hand, we will be ready to really upgrade to the Information Age. Just like Wikipedia allowed the advent of Artificial Intelligence, our crowdsourcing dental database can open the doors to more efficient and cheaper solutions to serve the public.

I choose to honour my oath to serve the public by embracing progress and working to give them what they want: better care, more accessibility, and affordability. What about you? Will you join me in making dentistry more accessible, more human, and closer to the people we swore to serve?

"Needed changes will come from technological advancement, especially in the medical field."

Dr. Bak Nguyen

This is **LEADERSHIP volume 1, CHANGING THE WORLD FROM A DENTAL CHAIR** presented by ALPHA DENTISTRY. Welcome to the Alphas.

Dr. BAK NGUYEN

CONCLUSION

By Dr. BAK NGUYEN

What a journey this was. It started 8 months ago, as Mahsa wanted for us to start writing our book on leadership. 8 months later, we are 10 international dental leaders joining forces to share our vision about how our profession is broken, and yet, we are not giving up on it! If anything, it ignited even more passion in each of us to care for the wounds and void of the dental industry.

68,561 words so far! This is scary! How did we write so much?! Is our profession that broken? Well, yes. To rebuild it, we need vision, we need hope, we need to stop denying, we need to drop EGO, we need to embrace technology, we need to remind ourselves of whom we serve, we need all of us united! Our profession is changing, people's patience is growing thin and the time for diagnostic is over. We need action, we need to try different avenues and to readjust from there.

To hide behind the past, the average, the norms is not good enough, not anymore! And what average did you have in mind? I hope that it wasn't how high we score on the depression board!

Our profession is changing. Just like democracy is shaping the society of tomorrow, our profession is gaining more and more popularity with our female colleagues. In some countries, the majority of dentists are women. That's a reality that we must incorporate into our vision and leadership.

I am a male and an Alpha, but it would be a huge oversight to not recognize the traits of our profession by 2023. Actually, we have so much to fix to keep building on denial, past mistakes, and oversight. I had that discussion with Gurien. Well, to us, there is no male or female leadership, just problems and solutions. Masha, Katalin, Sandra, and Marilyn all mentioned how different it is for a woman to exercise our profession.

I won't argue with feminism and gender equality. What I will state is that, it is a well-established fact that women are composing the majority within our ranks. In democratic societies, that is a shift in power, in paradigm.

Don't get me wrong, I am a proud man. But as an Alpha, I don't want to be part of the problem, the next one either. Thank you for allowing me to clarify the status of our profession, especially after reviewing each word of this book, each taught shared by the inspiring leaders who joined forces to rebuild our profession.

"No one can stand in the way of progress for long and hope for a win."
Dr. Bak Nguyen

Well, to face change and to catch-up, we need the right mindset, one of openness, one with our heart and eye open to stop the denials, one that will stop hiding behind the security of past perfection, of past traditions, of the fading past. If we need to change, we must break from our safety margin and security. Actually, I think that we cover that part in depth: it is either we change, drastically, or we will get replaced with better and cheaper, and much sooner than we can accept.

So more than a mindset, we also need to network and work together, as an industry. Dentists, hygienists, team members, supporting staff, from the front desk to marketing, even dental companies and universities. The silo mentality and tunnel vision have crippled our profession for too long. It is time for a change!

"I don't care who is right, for as long one of us is!"
Dr. Bak Nguyen

We need to change the core of our mindset to come together and to unite, not to be left behind. To change, we need all of us. But that won't be enough. We will need a great lever to change the entitlements and rusted ways. We will need a technological paradox.

Well, we got COVID to wake us with a cold shower. That can be a curse or a blessing, it will be for you to decide. But now that we are awake and networking, as Professor Nagy clearly stated, will you go back to your corner, blindsided? Change is not something our profession likes or even accepts. Much resistance will arise.

Well, we are smart people, aren't we? COVID proved that we are not that important to the medical field! The stats say that we are not happy and the public, well, let's not go there… And recent history showed us how eager the public and the governing bodies are ease with the idea to replace us with cheaper alternatives, more flexible solutions… Well, if this is not a standard yet, it will, be if we do not change our approach.

Look around you. In the midst of such a tormented world, between COVID, the wars, the shortage of staff, and our leadership crisis, we are privileged to witness a shift in technology: the free flow of information and the rapid evolution of artificial intelligence. This will change everything in a matter of years, even months. How much longer will you stand on the side complaining about the past?

This is **LEADERSHIP volume 1, CHANGING THE WORLD FROM A DENTAL CHAIR** presented by ALPHA DENTISTRY. Welcome to the Alphas.

Dr. BAK NGUYEN

ANNEX

GLOSSARY OF Dr. BAK's LIBRARY

1

REINVENT YOURSELF FROM ANY CRISIS

BY Dr. BAK NGUYEN

1SELF is about reinventing yourself to rise from any crisis. Written in the midst of the COVID war, now more than ever, we need hope and the know-how to bridge the future. More than just the journey of Dr. Bak, this time, Dr. Bak is sharing his journey with mentors and people who built part of the world as we know it. Interviewed in this book, CHRISTIAN TRUDEAU, former CEO and FOUNDER of BCE EMERGIS (BELL CANADA), he also digitalized the Montreal Stock Exchange. RON KLEIN, American Innovator, inventor of the magnetic stripe of the credit card, of MLS (Multi-listing services) and the man who digitalized WALL STREET bonds markets.ANDRE CHATELAIN, former first vice-president of the MOVEMENT DESJARDINS. Dr. JEAN DE SERRES, former CEO of HEMA QUEBEC. These men created billions in values and have changed our lives, even without us knowing. They all come together to share their experiences and knowledge to empower each and everyone to emerge stronger from this crisis, from any crisis.

A

AI - TO COME
HOW TO LEVERAGE ARTIFICIAL INTELLIGENCE FOR SOCIAL MEDIA
BY Dr. BAK NGUYEN & JAMES STEPHAN-USYPCHUK

In AI HOW TO LEVERAGE ARTIFICIAL INTELLIGENCE FOR SOCIAL MEDIA, Dr. Bak is teaming up with AI pioneer James Stephan-Usypchuk at the forefront of technology to understand and to leverage AI to ease the rise of leaders and entrepreneurs. As the AGE OF AI has begun to set, many are still wondering how to react. Should we feel concerned and threaten to be replaced? Or should we embrace the technology for a meteorite rise? Dr. Bak is sharing his experience and views on the matter as he chose to incorporate AI into his daily work. This book is not solely about the merit or danger of AI but how to use it to rise, with more ease. AI - HOW TO LEVERAGE ARTIFICIAL INTELLIGENCE the new frontier in Dr. Bak's evolution as he continues his YES path, welcoming the new and adapting as he moves forward. Welcome to the Alphas.

AFTERMATH -063
BUSINESS AFTER THE GREAT PAUSE
BY Dr. BAK NGUYEN & Dr. ERIC LACOSTE

In AFTERMATH, Dr. Bak joins forces with Community leader and philanthrope Dr. Eric Lacoste. Two powerful minds and forces of nature in the reaction to the worst economic meltdown in modern times. We are all victims of the CORONA virus. Both just like humans have learnt to adapt to survive, so is our economy. Most business structures and management philosophies are inherited from the age of industrialization and beyond. COVID-19 has shot down the world economy for months. At the time of the AFTERMATH, the truth is many corporations and organizations will either have to upgrade to the INFORMATION AGE or disappear. More than the INFORMATION upgrade, the era of SOCIAL MEDIA and the MILLENNIALS are driving a revolution in the core philosophy of all organizations. Profit is not king anymore, support is. In this time and age where a teenager with a social account can compete with the million dollars PR firm, social implication is now the new cornerstone. Those who will adapt will prevail and prosper, while the resistance and old guards will soon be forgotten as fossils of a past era.

ALPHA DENTISTRY vol. 1 -104
DIGITAL ORTHODONTIC FAQ

BY Dr. BAK NGUYEN

In ALPHA DENTISTRY, DIGITAL ORTHODONTICS FAQ, Dr. Bak is looking to democratize the science of dentistry, starting with orthodontics. In a word, he is sharing everything a patient needs to know on the matter in FAQ form. In order to make the knowledge complete and universal, Dr. Bak has invited Alpha Dentists from all around the world to join in and answer the same question. With Alpha Dentists from America and Europe, ALPHA DENTISTRY is the first effort to create a universal knowledge in the field of dentistry, starting with orthodontics. ALPHA DENTISTRY, DIGITAL ORTHODONTICS FAQ is in response to the COVID crisis, the shortage of staff crisis, and the effort to unify dentistry to the Information Age, as discussed in RELEVANCY and COVIDCONOMICS, THE DENTAL INDUSTRY.

ALPHA DENTISTRY vol. 1 -109
DIGITAL ORTHODONTIC FAQ ASSEMBLED EDITION

🇨🇦 CANADA 🇩🇪 GERMANY 🇮🇳 INDIA 🇺🇸 USA 🇪🇸 SPAIN
BY Dr. BAK NGUYEN, Dr. PAUL OUELLETTE, Dr. PAUL DOMINIQUE, Dr. MARIA KUNSTADTER, Dr. EDWARD J. ZUCKERBERG, Dr. MASHA KHAGHANI, Dr. SUJATA BASAWARAJ, Dr. ALVA AURORA, Dr. JUDITH BÄUMLER, and Dr. ASHISH GUPTA

In ALPHA DENTISTRY, DIGITAL ORTHODONTICS FAQ, Dr. Bak is democratizing the science of dentistry, starting with orthodontics. In a word, he is sharing everything a patient needs to know on the matter in FAQ form, simple words you'll understand.10 International Alpha Doctors, from USA, Spain, Germany, India, and Canada are joining forces to make the knowledge complete and universal. ALPHA DENTISTRY is the first effort to create a universal knowledge in the field of dentistry, this is the orthodontics volume. This is the most ambitious book project in the History of Dentistry. ALPHA DENTISTRY is in response to the COVID crisis, the shortage of staff crisis, and the effort to unify dentistry to the Information Age, as discussed in RELEVANCY and COVIDCONOMICS, THE DENTAL INDUSTRY.

ALPHA DENTISTRY vol. 1 -113
DIGITAL ORTHODONTIC FAQ INTERNATIONAL EDITION

ENGLISH FRENCH GERMAN HINDI SPANISH
BY Dr. BAK NGUYEN, Dr. PAUL OUELLETTE, Dr. PAUL DOMINIQUE, Dr. MARIA KUNSTADTER, Dr. EDWARD J. ZUCKERBERG, Dr. MASHA KHAGHANI, Dr. SUJATA BASAWARAJ, Dr. ALVA AURORA, Dr. JUDITH BÄUMLER, and Dr. ASHISH GUPTA

In ALPHA DENTISTRY, DIGITAL ORTHODONTICS FAQ, Dr. Bak is democratizing the science of dentistry, starting with orthodontics. In a word, he is sharing everything a patient needs to know on the matter in FAQ form, simple words you'll understand.10 International Alpha Doctors, from USA, Spain, Germany, India, and Canada are joining forces to make the knowledge complete and universal. ALPHA DENTISTRY is the first effort to create a universal knowledge in the field of dentistry, this is the orthodontics volume. This is the most ambitious book project in the History of Dentistry. ALPHA DENTISTRY is in response to the COVID crisis, the shortage of staff crisis, and the effort to unify dentistry to the Information Age, as discussed in RELEVANCY and COVIDCONOMICS, THE DENTAL INDUSTRY.

ALPHA DENTISTRY vol. 2 -127
IMPLANTOLOGY FAQ ASSEMBLED EDITION

ALBANIA BRAZIL CANADA INDIA MALAYSIA PORTUGAL SPAIN USA
BY Dr. BAK NGUYEN, Dr. ERIC LACOSTE , Dr. PRETINDER SINGH, Dr. SANDEEP SINGH, Dr. ERIC PULVER, Dr. ARASH HAKHAMIAN, Dr. MAHSA KHAGHANI, Dr. BENNETE FERNANDES, Dr. RAQUEL ZITA GOMES, Dr. SANDRA FABIANO and Dr. GURIEN DEMIRAQI

In ALPHA DENTISTRY, IMPLANTOLOGY FAQ, Dr. Bak is democratizing the science of dentistry, with the sub-specialty of IMPLANTOLOGY, which expertise is shared between Periodontists, Oral Surgeons and Dentists. In a word, he is sharing everything a patient needs to know on the matter in FAQ form, simple words you'll understand.11 International Alpha Doctors, from USA, India, Portugal, Spain, Brazil, Malaysia, Albania and Canada are joining forces to make the knowledge complete and universal. ALPHA DENTISTRY is the first effort to create a universal knowledge in the field of dentistry, this is the IMPLANTOLOGY volume. This is the most ambitious book project in the History of Dentistry. The whole book is covered in English and each author with a different native tongue is also covering their chapters in their native language. ALPHA DENTISTRY is in response to the COVID crisis, the shortage of staff crisis, and the effort to unify dentistry to the Information Age, as discussed in RELEVANCY and COVIDCONOMICS, THE DENTAL INDUSTRY.

ALPHA DENTISTRY vol. 2 -128
IMPLANTOLOGY FAQ INTERNATIONAL EDITION

ALBANIAN ENGLISH FRANÇAIS GERMAN HINDI ITALIAN KANNADA MALAY MANDARIN PORTUGUESE SPANISH

BY Dr. BAK NGUYEN, Dr. ERIC LACOSTE , Dr. PRETINDER SINGH, Dr. SANDEEP SINGH, Dr. ERIC PULVER, Dr. ARASH HAKHAMIAN, Dr. MAHSA KHAGHANI, Dr. BENNETE FERNANDES, Dr. RAQUEL ZITA GOMES, Dr. SANDRA FABIANO and Dr. GURIEN DEMIRAQI

In ALPHA DENTISTRY, IMPLANTOLOGY FAQ, Dr. Bak is democratizing the science of dentistry, with the sub-specialty of IMPLANTOLOGY, which expertise is shared between Periodontists, Oral Surgeons and Dentists. In a word, he is sharing everything a patient needs to know on the matter in FAQ form, simple words you'll understand.11 International Alpha Doctors, from USA, India, Portugal, Spain, Brazil, Malaysia, Albania and Canada are joining forces to make the knowledge complete and universal. ALPHA DENTISTRY is the first effort to create a universal knowledge in the field of dentistry, this is the IMPLANTOLOGY volume. This is the most ambitious book project in the History of Dentistry. The whole book is covered in English and each author with a different native tongue is also covering their chapters in their native language. ALPHA DENTISTRY is in response to the COVID crisis, the shortage of staff crisis, and the effort to unify dentistry to the Information Age, as discussed in RELEVANCY and COVIDCONOMICS, THE DENTAL INDUSTRY.

ALPHA DENTISTRY vol. 3 -131
PAEDIATRIC FAQ ASSEMBLED EDITION

CANADA EGYPT GERMANY ITALY MALTA PERU UNITED ARAB EMIRATES USA

BY Dr. BAK NGUYEN, Dr. PAUL DOMINIQUE, Dr. RICHARD SIMPSON, Dr. AURORA ALVA, Dr. NOUR AMMAR, Dr. AILIN CABRERA-MATTA, Dr. NIDHI TANEJA, Dr. PIERLUIGI PELAGALLI, Dr. PRRIYA PORWAL

In ALPHA DENTISTRY, PAEDIATRIC FAQ, Dr. Bak is democratizing the science of dentistry, this time, focusing on children. From all of dentistry, this is the kindest and most humane specialty of DENTISTRY. From the USA to Germany, Peru to Egypt and Canada, experts around the world are joining this collaborative effort welcome, reassure, and empower parents and kids on their quest to a healthy mouth. ALPHA DENTISTRY is the first effort to create a universal knowledge in the field of dentistry, this is the PAEDIATRIC volume. This is the most ambitious book project in the History of Dentistry. The whole book is covered in English and each author with a different native tongue is also covering their chapters in their native language. ALPHA DENTISTRY is in response to the COVID crisis, the shortage of staff crisis, and the effort to unify dentistry to the Information Age, as discussed in RELEVANCY and COVIDCONOMICS, THE DENTAL INDUSTRY.

ALPHA DENTISTRY vol. 3 -132
PAEDIATRIC FAQ INTERNATIONAL EDITION

ENGLISH ARABIC FRANÇAIS ITALIAN MALTESE SPANISH
BY Dr. BAK NGUYEN, Dr. PAUL DOMINIQUE, Dr. RICHARD SIMPSON, Dr. AURORA ALVA, Dr. NOUR AMMAR, Dr. AILIN CABRERA-MATTA, Dr. NIDHI TANEJA, Dr. PIERLUIGI PELAGALLI, Dr. PRRIYA PORWAL

In ALPHA DENTISTRY, PAEDIATRIC FAQ, Dr. Bak is democratizing the science of dentistry, this time, focusing on children. From all of dentistry, this is the kindest and most humane specialty of DENTISTRY. From the USA to Germany, Peru to Egypt and Canada, experts around the world are joining this collaborative effort welcome, reassure, and empower parents and kids on their quest to a healthy mouth. ALPHA DENTISTRY is the first effort to create a universal knowledge in the field of dentistry, this is the PAEDIATRIC volume. This is the most ambitious book project in the History of Dentistry. The whole book is covered in English and each author with a different native tongue is also covering their chapters in their native language. ALPHA DENTISTRY is in response to the COVID crisis, the shortage of staff crisis, and the effort to unify dentistry to the Information Age, as discussed in RELEVANCY and COVIDCONOMICS, THE DENTAL INDUSTRY.

ALPHA DENTISTRY vol. 4 -135
PAEDIATRIC DENTISTRY FAQ ASSEMBLED EDITION

ALBANIA AUSTRALIA CANADA GERMANY INDIA IRAN MALAYSIA SPAIN USA
BY Dr. BAK NGUYEN, Dr. ERIC LACOSTE, Dr. MAZIAR SHAHZAD DOWLATSHAHI, Dr. BENNETE FERNANDES, Dr. MEENU BHASIN, Dr. HASTEE BHANUSHALI, Dr. ROBERT M. PICK, Dr. AMIN MOTAMEDI, Dr. TIHANA DIVNIC-RESNIK, Dr. ARNE VON STERNHEIM, Dr. FERNANDO ARPÓN MORENO and Dr. GURIEN DEMIRAQI

In ALPHA DENTISTRY, PERIODONTICS FAQ, Dr. Bak is democratizing the science of dentistry, with the sub-specialty of PERIODONTOLOGY, which expertise is shared between Periodontists, Oral Surgeons and Dentists. In a word, he is sharing everything a patient needs to know on the matter in FAQ form, simple words you'll understand.11 International Alpha Doctors, from the USA, India, Australia, Iran, Malaysia, Albania and Canada are joining forces to make the knowledge complete and universal. ALPHA DENTISTRY is the first effort to create a universal knowledge in the field of dentistry, this is the PERIODONTICS volume. This is the most ambitious book project in the History of Dentistry. The whole book is covered in English and each author with a different native tongue is also covering their chapters in their native language. ALPHA DENTISTRY is in response to the COVID crisis, the shortage of staff crisis, and the effort to unify dentistry to the Information Age, as discussed in RELEVANCY and COVIDCONOMICS, THE DENTAL INDUSTRY.

ALPHA DENTISTRY vol. 4 -136
PAEDIATRIC DENTISTRY FAQ INTERNATIONAL EDITION

ENGLISH FRENCH GERMAN HINDI ITALIAN MANDARIN MALAY ARABIC SPANISH SHQIP

BY Dr. BAK NGUYEN, Dr. ERIC LACOSTE, Dr. MAZIAR SHAHZAD DOWLATSHAHI, Dr. BENNETE FERNANDES, Dr. MEENU BHASIN, Dr. HASTEE BHANUSHALI, Dr. ROBERT M. PICK, Dr. AMIN MOTAMEDI, Dr. TIHANA DIVNIC-RESNIK, Dr. ARNE VON STERNHEIM, Dr. FERNANDO ARPÓN MORENO and Dr. GURIEN DEMIRAQI

In ALPHA DENTISTRY, PERIODONTICS FAQ, Dr. Bak is democratizing the science of dentistry, with the sub-specialty of PERIODONTOLOGY, which expertise is shared between Periodontists, Oral Surgeons and Dentists. In a word, he is sharing everything a patient needs to know on the matter in FAQ form, simple words you'll understand.11 International Alpha Doctors, from the USA, India, Germany, Spain, Australia, Iran, Malaysia, Albania and Canada are joining forces to make the knowledge complete and universal. ALPHA DENTISTRY is the first effort to create a universal knowledge in the field of dentistry, this is the PERIODONTICS volume. This is the most ambitious book project in the History of Dentistry. The whole book is covered in English and each author with a different native tongue is also covering their chapters in their native language. ALPHA DENTISTRY is in response to the COVID crisis, the shortage of staff crisis, and the effort to unify dentistry to the Information Age, as discussed in RELEVANCY and COVIDCONOMICS, THE DENTAL INDUSTRY.

ALPHA DENTISTRY vol. 5 -137
PAEDIATRIC DENTISTRY FAQ ASSEMBLED EDITION

AUSTRALIA CANADA FRANCE LITHUANIA PERU TURKEY UKRAINE USA

BY Dr. BAK NGUYEN, Dr. JULIO REYNAFARJE, Dr. LINA DUSEVIČIŪTĖ, Dr. NAZARIY MYKHAYLYUK, Dr. CLAUDE MOUAFO, Dr. MANOJ RAJAN, Dr. LOUIS KAUFMAN, Dr. LILIAN SHI and Dr. YASEMIN OZKAN

In ALPHA DENTISTRY, COSMETIC DENTISTRY FAQ, Dr. Bak is democratizing the science of dentistry, with the sub-specialty of COSMETIC DENTISTRY, which expertise is shared between Prosthodontists and Dentists. In a word, he is sharing everything a patient needs to know on the matter in FAQ form, simple words you'll understand. International Alpha Doctors, from the USA, France, Peru, Lithuania, Ukraine, Australia, Turkey and Canada are joining forces to make the knowledge complete and universal.ALPHA DENTISTRY is the first effort to create a universal knowledge in the field of dentistry, this is the COSMETIC DENTISTRY volume. This is the most ambitious book project in the History of Dentistry. The whole book is covered in English and each author with a different native tongue is also covering their chapters in their native language. ALPHA DENTISTRY is in response to the COVID crisis, the shortage of staff crisis, and the effort to unify dentistry to the Information Age, as discussed in RELEVANCY and COVIDCONOMICS, THE DENTAL INDUSTRY.

ALPHA DENTISTRY vol. 5 138
PAEDIATRIC DENTISTRY FAQ INTERNATIONAL EDITION

ENGLISH ARABIC FRENCH LITHUANIAN SPANISH UKRAINIAN
BY Dr. BAK NGUYEN, Dr. JULIO REYNAFARJE, Dr. LINA DUSEVIČIŪTĖ, Dr. NAZARIY MYKHAYLYUK, Dr. CLAUDE MOUAFO, Dr. MANOJ RAJAN, Dr. LOUIS KAUFMAN, Dr. LILIAN SHI and Dr. YASEMIN OZKAN

In ALPHA DENTISTRY, COSMETIC DENTISTRY FAQ, Dr. Bak is democratizing the science of dentistry, with the sub-specialty of COSMETIC DENTISTRY, which expertise is shared between Prosthodontists and Dentists. In a word, he is sharing everything a patient needs to know on the matter in FAQ form, simple words you'll understand. International Alpha Doctors, from the USA, France, Peru, Lithuania, Ukraine, Australia, Turkey and Canada are joining forces to make the knowledge complete and universal.ALPHA DENTISTRY is the first effort to create a universal knowledge in the field of dentistry, this is the COSMETIC DENTISTRY volume. This is the most ambitious book project in the History of Dentistry. The whole book is covered in English and each author with a different native tongue is also covering their chapters in their native language. ALPHA DENTISTRY is in response to the COVID crisis, the shortage of staff crisis, and the effort to unify dentistry to the Information Age, as discussed in RELEVANCY and COVIDCONOMICS, THE DENTAL INDUSTRY.

ALPHA LADDERS 075
CAPTAIN OF YOUR DESTINY
BY Dr. BAK NGUYEN & JONAS DIOP

In ALPHA LADDERS, Dr. Bak is sharing his private conversation and board meetings with 2 of his trusted lieutenants, strategist Jonas Diop and international Counsellor, Brenda Garcia. As both Dr. Bak and ALPHA brands are gaining in popularity and traction, it was time to get the movement to the next level. Now, it's about building a community and helping everyone willing to become ALPHAS to find their powers. Dr. Bak is a natural recruiter of ALPHAS and peers. He also spent the last 20 years plus, training and mentoring proteges. Now comes the time to empower more and more proteges to become ALPHAS. ALPHAS LADDERS is the journey of how Dr. Bak went from a product of Conformity to rise into a force of Nature, known as a kind tornado. In ALPHA LADDERS Jonas pushed Dr. Bak to retrace each of the steps of his awakening, steps that we can break down and reproduce for ourselves. The goal is to empower each willing individual to become the ultimate Captain of his or her destiny, and to do it, again and again. Welcome to the Alphas.

ALPHA LADDERS 2 -081
SHAPING LEADERS AND ACHIEVERS
BY Dr. BAK NGUYEN & BRENDA GARCIA

In ALPHA LADDERS 2, Dr. Bak is sharing the second part of his private conversation and board meetings with his trusted lieutenants. This time it is with international Counsellor, Brenda Garcia that the dialogue is taking place. In this second tome, the journey is taken to the next level. If the first tome was about the WHYs and the HOWs at an individual level, this tome is about the WHYs and the HOWs at the societal level. Through the lens of her background in international relations and diplomacy, Brenda now has the mission to help Dr. Bak establish structures, not only for his emerging organization and legacy, THE ALPHAS, but to also inspire all the other leaders and structures of our society. To do this, Brenda is taking Dr. Bak on an anthropological, sociological and philosophical journey to revisit different historical key moments in various fields and eras, going as far back as ancient Greece at the dawn of democracy, all the way to the golden era of modern multilateralism embodied by the UN structure. Learning from the legacies of prominent figures going from Plato to Ban Ki-Moon, Martin Luther King or Nelson Mandela, to Machiavelli, Marx and Simone de Beauvoir, Brenda and Dr. Bak are attempting to grasp the essence of structure and hierarchy, their goal being to empower each willing individual to become the ultimate Captain of their success, to climb up the ladders no matter how high it is, and to build their legacy one step at a time.

ALPHA MASTERMIND vol. 1 -116
THE SUPERHERO'S SYNDROME
BY Dr. BAK NGUYEN

ALPHA MASTERMIND, THE SUPER HERO'S SYNDROME, is not a superhero book, but it is the tale of every leader, entrepreneur, and everyday hero facing their destiny and entourage. It uncovers how society sees our best elements and expects from them. It covers how family and friends feel and why they act as they do. But most importantly, it covers how Alphas can emerge unscathed from their growth to uncover their true powers and purpose. A veteran agent of change and difference maker, Dr. Bak is sharing his experience and secret of why and how surfing through family and society pressure without revolting and without kneeling. THE SUPERHERO'S SYNDROME is the first volume inspired by the MASTERMINDS sessions as Dr. Bak is mentoring Alpha apprentices. The superhero's syndrome came to the table as Alphas are struggling to fit in society, to keep their values and generosity while facing so much negativity all around. Welcome to the Alphas.

ALPHA MASTERMIND vol. 2 -117
SUPERCHARGING MOMENTUM
BY Dr. BAK NGUYEN

ALPHA MASTERMIND, SUPERCHARGING MOMENTUM, is what is discussed on the Alphas' Round Table. Entrepreneurs, Professional Athletes, Coaches, they are all rising from their passion and momentum. To start was the first ACT. It wasn't easy but they did. Now as a FOOTBALL star, what can be next, not to fall as a HAS BEEN? You wrote your first book, what is next? What comes next after 100 books?There are so many paths to finding your powers but there is only one that I know that will keep feeding them: MOMENTUM. If discovering your powers and purposes was a great journey, the sequel to that story is a much harder one to write, to walk, to thrive from. In every story, the hero needs to rise and to grow. How can one grow even more? SUPERCHARGING MOMENTUM is the 2nd volume inspired by the MASTERMINDS sessions as Dr. Bak is mentoring Alpha apprentices. Dr. Bak is not teaching, he is sharing what he faces and does to write his next life chapter, renewing and reinventing himself again and again. Welcome to the Alphas.

ALPHA MASTERMIND vol. 3 -118
RIDING DESTINY
BY Dr. BAK NGUYEN

In ALPHA MASTERMIND, RIDING DESTINY, Dr. Bak is taking you and his apprentices on the quest of rising. It will be for each to find their purpose and destiny, but the way leading there will be eased with Dr. Bak's guidance. To discover power was only the beginning, to yield power was a preparation journey, now it is about rendering power into a stream of ripple effect. "KNOW YOURSELF, KNOW THE OTHER, AND ONLY THEN, DEAL." - Dr. BAK. Well, the 2 first volumes were about knowing oneself, this one is about knowing the other and to start dealing. Once one finds power, it is barely the beginning of his or her quest. The process is not an easy one, going through separation, rejection, and denial. Then, there will be encounters of a new kind, those liberating instead of attaching.RIDING DESTINY, is the third volume inspired by the MASTERMINDS sessions as Dr. Bak is mentoring Alpha apprentices. This is about ROI on the energy invested and the one generated. Welcome to the Alphas.

AMONGST THE ALPHAS -058

BY Dr. BAK NGUYEN, with Dr. MARIA KUNSTADTER, Dr. PAUL OUELLETTE and Dr. JEREMY KRELL

In AMONGST THE ALPHAS, Dr. Bak opens the blueprint of the next level with the hope that everyone can be better, bigger, and wiser, but above all, a philosophy of Life that if, well applied, can bring inspiration to life. The Alphas rose in the midst of the COVID war as an International Collaboration to empower individuals to rise from the global crisis. Joining Dr. Bak are some of the world thinkers and achievers, the Alphas. Doctors, business people, thinkers, achievers, and influencers, are coming together to define what is an Alpha and his or her role, making the world a better place. This isn't the American dream, it is the human dream, one that can help you make History. Joining Dr. Bak are 3 Alpha authors, Dr. Maria Kunstadter, Dr. Paul Ouellette and Dr. Jeremy Krell. This book started with questions from coach Jonas Diop. Welcome to the Alphas.

AMONGST THE ALPHAS vol.2 -059
ON THE OTHER SIDE

BY Dr. BAK NGUYEN with Dr. JULIO REYNAFARJE, Dr. LINA DUSEVICIUTE and Dr. DUC-MINH LAM-DO

In AMONGST THE ALPHAS 2, Dr. Bak continues to explore the meaning of what it is to be an Alpha and how to act amongst Alphas, because as the saying taught us: alone one goes fast, together we go far. Some people see the problem. Some people look at the problem, some people created the problem. Some people leverage the problem into solutions and opportunities. Well, all of those people are Alphas. Networking and leveraging one another, their powers and reach are beyond measure. And one will keep the other in line too. Joining Dr. Bak are 3 Alphas from around the world coming together to share and collaborate, Dr. DUSEVICIUTE, Dr. LAM-DO and Dr. REYNAFARJE. This isn't the American dream, it is the human dream, one that can help you make History. Welcome to the Alphas.

APPRENTICESHIP -134
BY Dr. BAK NGUYEN & COACH MEL

APPRENTICESHIP, THE EMPOWERMENT OF POWER is the mirror of the conversation between a mentor and his apprentice. If in the first tome, MENTORSHIP, we followed the perspective of the mentor, in this tome, we are looking at the evolution from the apprentice's experience. The same image reflected through the mirror can be so different. Just as life is, reality lies in the eye of the beholder. In other words, there is no truth, just different perspectives with which, each makes their own reality. Following the conversation between Dr. Bak and Coach Mel, APPRENTICESHIP allows to see both perspectives, to live and feel both experiences and to leverage the experience of every end of the synergy. APPRENTICESHIP, THE EMPOWERMENT OF POWER is the story of an apprentice walking in the trails of her mentor while looking to beat him to honouring him. It is a journey of healing, of acceptance, of respect, and one of rising. This is the conversation between Dr. Bak and Coach Mel, on her path to setting the next world record mark in literature, beating her mentor. It is the universal dynamic of every mentor-apprentice synergy. Welcome to the Alphas.

AU PAYS DES PAPAS -106
BY Dr. BAK NGUYEN & WILLIAM BAK

On ne nait pas papa. On le devient. Dans sa quête d'être le meilleur papa possible pour William, Dr. Bak monte au pays des papas avec William à la recherche du papa parfait. Comme pour tout dans la vie, il doit exister une recette pour faire des papas parfaits. AU PAYS DES PAPAS est le récit des souvenirs des papas que Dr. Bak a croisé avant, alors et après qu'il soit devenu papa lui aussi. Une histoire drôle et innocente pour un Noël magique, ceci est la nouvelle aventure de William et de son papa, le Dr. Bak. Entre les livres de poulet, LEGENDS OF DESTINY et les des livres parentaux de Dr. Bak, AU PAYS DES PAPAS nous amène dans le monde magique de ces êtres magiques qui forgent des rêves, des vies et des destins.

AU PAYS DES PAPAS 2 -108
BY Dr. BAK NGUYEN & WILLIAM BAK

On ne nait pas papa, ça on le sait après le premier voyage AU PAYS DES PAPAS. Suite à leur première expédition, Dr. Bak et William ont compris qu'il n'y a pas de papas parfaits ni de recette pour faire des papas parfaits. Pourtant, les papas parfaits existent! Dans ce 2e récit

AU PAYS DES PAPAS, William revient avec son papa, Dr. Bak, mais cette fois, c'est William qui dirige l'expédition. Même s'il n'existe pas de recette pour faire des papas parfaits, il doit toutefois exister des façons de rendre son papa meilleur, version 2.0! C'est la nouvelle quête de William et du Dr. Bak, à la recherche de la mise-à-jour parfaite pour le meilleur papa 2.0 possible! William est déterminé à tout pour trouver la recette cette fois-ci! AU PAYS DES PAPAS 2 est le nouveau récit des aventures père-fils du Dr. Bak et de William Bak, après AU PAYS DES PAPAS 1, les livres de poulets, LEGENDS OF DESTINY et les BOOKS OF LEGENDS.

B

BOOTCAMP ·071
BOOKS TO REWRITE MINDSETS INTO WINNING STATES OF MIND
BY Dr. BAK NGUYEN

In BOOTCAMP 8 BOOKS TO REWRITE MINDSETS INTO WINNING STATES OF MIND, Dr. Bak is taking you into his past, before the visionary entrepreneur, before the world records, before the Industry's disruptor status. Here are 8 of the books that changed Dr. Bak's thinking and, therefore, reset his evolution into the course we now know him for. BOOTCAMP: 8 BOOKS TO REWRITE MINDSETS INTO WINNING STATES OF MIND, is a Bootcamp of 8 weeks for anyone looking to experience Dr. Bak's training to become THE Dr. BAK you came to know and love. This book will summarize how each title changed Dr. Bak's mindset into a state of mind and how he applied that to rewrite his destiny. 8 books to read, that's 8 weeks of Bootcamp to access the power of your MIND and your WILL. Are you ready for a change?

BRANDING 044
BALANCING STRATEGY AND EMOTIONS
BY Dr. BAK NGUYEN

BRANDING is communication to its most powerful state. Branding is not just about communicating anymore but about making a promise, about establishing a relationship, and about generating an emotion. More than once, Dr. Bak proved himself to be a master, communicating and branding his ideas into flags attracting interest and influence, nationally and internationally. In BRANDING, Dr. Bak shares a very unique and personal journey, branding Dr. Bak. How does he go from Dr. Nguyen, a loved and respected dentist to becoming Dr. Bak, a world anchor hosting THE ALPHAS in the medical and financial world? More than a personal journey, BRANDING helps to break down the steps to elevate someone with nothing else but the force of his or her spirit. Welcome to the Alphas.

C

CHANGING THE WORLD FROM A DENTAL CHAIR 007
BY Dr. BAK NGUYEN

Since he has received the EY's nomination for entrepreneur of the year for his startup Mdex & Co, Dr. Bak Nguyen has pushed the opportunity to the next level. Speaker, author, and businessman, Dr. Bak is a true entrepreneur and industries' disruptor. To compensate for the startup's status of Mdex & Co, he challenged himself to write a book based on the EY's questionnaire to share an in-depth vision of his company. With "Changing the World from a dental chair" Dr. Bak is sharing his thought process and philosophy to his approach to the industry. Not looking to revolutionize but rather to empower, he became, despite himself, an industries disruptor: an entrepreneur who has established a new benchmark. Dr. Bak Nguyen is a cosmetic dentist and visionary businessman who won the GRAND HOMAGE prize of "LYS de la Diversité" 2016, for his contribution as a citizen and entrepreneur in the community. He also holds recognitions from the Canadian Parliament and the Canadian Senate. In 2003, he founded Mdex, a dental company upon which in 2018, he launched the most ambitious private endeavour to reform the dental industry, Canada-wide. He wrote seven books covering ENTREPRENEURSHIP, LEADERSHIP, QUEST of IDENTITY, and now, PROFESSION HEALTH. Philosopher, he has close to his heart the quest of happiness of the people surrounding him, patients, and colleagues alike. Those projects have allowed Dr. Nguyen to attract interest from the international and diplomatic community and he is now the centre of a global discussion on the wellbeing and the future of the health profession. It is in that matter that he shares with you his thoughts and encourages the health community to share their own stories.

CHAMPION MINDSET -039
LEARNING TO WIN
BY Dr. BAK NGUYEN & CHRISTOPHE MULUMBA

CHAMPION MINDSET is the encounter of the business world and the professional sports world. Industries' Disruptor Dr. BAK NGUYEN shares his wisdom and views with the HAMMER, CFL Football Star, Edmonton's Eskimos CHRISTOPHE MULUMBA on how to leverage the champion mindset to create successful entrepreneurs. Writing and challenging each other, they discovered the parallels and the difference of both worlds, but mainly, the recipe for leveraging from one to succeed in the other, from champions and entrepreneurs to WINNERS. Build and score your millions, it is a matter of mindset! This is CHAMPION MINDSET.

COMMENT ÉCRIRE UN LIVRE EN 30 JOURS -102
PAR Dr. BAK NGUYEN

Dans COMMENT ÉCRIRE UN LIVRE EN 30 JOURS, après plus de 100 livres écrits en 4 ans, le Dr Bak revisite son premier succès, le livre dans lequel il a partagé son art et sa structure d'écriture de livres. Encore et encore, le Dr Bak a prouvé que non seulement le contenu est important, mais ce sont la structure et le processus qui rendent les livres. L'inspiration n'est que le début. Si vous envisagez d'écrire votre premier livre, ceci est votre chance. Si vous y pensez, faites-le, et aussi vite que possible. Écrire votre premier livre vous libérera de votre passé et vous ouvrira les portes de votre avenir! Tout le monde a une histoire qui mérite d'être partagée! Par où commencer, comment passer le MUR DE L'INSPIRATION, quelles sont les techniques pour apporter de la profondeur à votre histoire, comment structurer votre chapitre, combien de chapitres, comment avoir un livre, en un mois? Voilà les réponses que vous trouverez dans COMMENT ÉCRIRE UN LIVRE EN 30 JOURS. Vous trouverez un trésor de sagesse, un mentor et surtout, une confiance renouvelée pour écrire, que ce soit, votre premier, deuxième ou même 10e livre. Au fait, le Dr. Bak a écrit ce livre et l'a fait publier en 6 jours. Bienvenu(e)s aux Alphas.

COMMENT ÉCRIRE 2 LIVRES EN 10 JOURS -115
Par WILLIAM & Dr. BAK NGUYEN

Dans COMMENT ÉCRIRE 2 LIVRES EN 10 JOURS, William Bak s'attaque au succès de son père, COMMENT ÉCRIRE UN LIVRE EN 30 JOURS. Cette fois-ci, père et fils font équipe pour vous partager l'art d'écrire de la fiction. Comme le titre le mentionne, William doit écrire ce livre et le suivant en 10 jours. Pour ne pas vous induire en erreur, écrire votre premier livre de fiction prendra plus que 10 jours. Cependant, les procédés contenus dans ce livre vous aideront à accélérer votre production et à porter votre créativité à des niveaux inégalés. William a 12 ans et déjà, il a signé 36 livres dont la plupart sont de la fiction. En ce sens, il est un vétéran auteur, un qui a connu les hauts et les bas du manque d'inspiration. Au côté de William, Dr. Bak se prête aussi au jeux de démolir son propre succès et le remplacer par une nouvelle marque. Père et fils, ils vous partagent leurs secrets et expérience à écrire un duo-choque depuis les derniers 4 ans. COMMENT ÉCRIRE 2 LIVRES EN 10 JOURS a commencé par une farce qui est rapidement devenu leur plus grand défi à ce jour, d'écrire 2 livres en 10 jours. Bienvenu(e)s aux Alphas.

COVIDCONOMIE -111
CONTRER L'INFLATION SANS TOUCHER LES TAUX D'INTÉRÊT
PAR Dr. BAK NGUYEN, ANDRÉ CHÂTEALAIN, TRANIE VO, FRANÇOIS DUFOUR, WILLIAM BAK

COVIDCONOMIE est l'ensemble des observations, analyses des phénomènes démographiques et économiques secondaires à la pandémie de la COVID-19. CONTRER L'INFLATION SANS TOUCHER LES TAUX D'INTÉRÊT, est la réflexion et plan macro des ALPHAS pour le CANADA et les ÉTATS-UNIS D'AMÉRIQUE dans un premier temps et un modèle économique pour l'ensemble des pays d'Occident.Joint par des leaders en finance et en économie, dont André Châtelain, ancien premier vice-président du MOUVEMENT DESJARDINS, le Dr. Bak met la table à des discussions inclusives et constructives pouvant changer le cours de l'Histoire dans l'intérêt des citoyens au quotidien.CONTRER L'INFLATION SANS TOUCHER LES TAUX D'INTÉRÊT, est un mémoire collectif des ALPHAS pour lutter contre l'inflation post-pandémique et éviter une récession internationale globale.

COVIDCONOMICS -112
TAMING INFLATION WITHOUT INCREASING INTEREST RATES
BY Dr. BAK NGUYEN, ANDRÉ CHÂTEALAIN, TRANIE VO, FRANÇOIS DUFOUR, WILLIAM BAK

COVIDCONOMICS, are the reflections, analysis and discussion of the ALPHAS, hosted by Dr. Bak to understand the demographic et economical trends post-COVID-19. TAMING INFLATION WITHOUT INCREASING INTEREST RATES is a macro plan by the ALPHAS for Canada and the USA which can inspire a new economical model for all of the Western worlds. Joined by leaders in finance as André Châtelain, former 1st Vice-President of the MOUVEMENT DESJARDINS, Dr. Bak is hosting an inclusive discussion to save our economy in these very troubled times as the country is still looking to get back on its feet from the Pandemic while wars are raging on multiple fronts. TAMING INFLATION WITHOUT INCREASING INTEREST RATES is our proposal to save the economy and our recovery from a global recession.

E

EMPOWERMENT -069
BY Dr. BAK NGUYEN

In EMPOWERMENT, Dr. Bak's 69th book, writing a book every 8 days for 8 weeks in a row to write the next world record of writing 72 books/36 months, Dr. Bak is taking a rest, sharing his inner feelings, inspiration, and motivation. Much more than his dairy, EMPOWERMENT is the key to walking in his footsteps and comprehending the process of an overachiever. Dr. Bak's helped and inspired countless people to find their voice, to live their dream, and to be the better version of themselves. Why is he sharing as much and keep sharing? Why is he going that fast, always further and further, why and how is he keeping his inspiration and momentum? Those are all the answers EMPOWERMENT will deliver to you. This book might be one of the fastest Dr. Bak has written, not because of time constraints but from inspiration, pure inspiration to share and to grow. There is always a dark side to each power, two faces to a coin. Well, this is the less prominent facet of Dr. Bak's Momentum and success, the road to his MINDSET.

F

FORCES OF NATURE ·015
FORGING THE CHARACTER OF WINNERS
BY Dr. BAK NGUYEN

In FORCES OF NATURE, Dr. Bak is giving his all. This is his 15 books written within 15 months. It is the end of a marathon to set the next world record. For the occasion, he wanted to end with a big bang! How about a book with all of his biggest challenges? In a Quest of Identity, a journey looking for his name and powers, Dr. Bak is borrowing myths and legends to make this journey universal. Yes, this is Dr. Bak's mythology. Demons, heroes and Gods, there are forces of Nature that we all meet on our way for our name. Some will scare us, some will fight us, and some will manipulate us. We can flee, we can hide, we can fight. What we do will define our next encounter and the one after. A tale of personal growth, a journey to find power and purpose, Dr. Bak is showing us the path to freedom, the Path of Life. Welcome to the Alphas.

H

HORIZON, BUILDING UP THE VISION -045
VOLUME ONE
BY Dr. BAK NGUYEN

Dr. Bak is opening up to your demand! Many of you are following Dr. Bak online and are asking to know more about his lifestyle. This is how he has chosen to respond: sharing his lifestyle as he travelled the world and what he learnt in each city to come to build his Mindset as a driver and a winner. Here are 10 destinations (over 69 that will be followed in the next volumes...) in which he shares his journey. New York, Quebec, Paris, Punta Cana, Monaco, Los Angeles, Nice, and Holguin, the journey happened over twenty years.

HORIZON, ON THE FOOTSTEP OF TITANS -048
VOLUME TWO
BY Dr. BAK NGUYEN

Dr. Bak is opening up to your demand! Many of you are following Dr. Bak online and are asking to know more about his lifestyle. This is how he has chosen to respond: sharing his lifestyle as he travelled the world and what he learnt in each city to come to build his Mindset as a driver and a winner. Here are 9 destinations (over 72 that will follow in the next volumes...) in which he shares his journey. Hong Kong, London, Rome, San Francisco, Anaheim, and more..., the journey happened over twenty years. Dr. Bak is sharing with you his feelings, impressions, and how they shaped his state of mind and character into Dr. Bak. From a dreamer to a driver and a builder, the journey started when he was 3. Wealth is a state of mind, and a state of mind is the basis of the drive. Find out about the mind of an Industry's disruptor.

Dr. Bak is back. From the midst of confinement, he remembers and writes about what life was, when travelling was a natural part of Life. It will come back. Now more than ever, we need to open both our hearts and minds to fight fear and intolerance. Writing from a time of crisis, he is sharing the magic and psychological effect of seeing the world and how it has shaped his mindset. Here are 9 other destinations (over 75) in which he shares his journey. Beijing, Key West, Madrid, Amsterdam, Marrakech and more…, the journey happened over twenty years.

In HOW TO BOOST YOUR CREATIVITY TO NEW HEIGHTS, Dr. Bak is sharing his secrets of creativity and insane production pace with the world. Up to lately, Dr. Bak shared his secrets about speed and momentum but never has he opened up about where he gets his inspiration, time and time again. To celebrate his new world record of writing 100 books in 4 years, Dr. Bak is joined by his proteges strategist Jonas Diop, international counsellor Brenda Garcia and prodigy William Bak for the writing of his secrets on creativity. Brenda, Jonas and William all have witnessed Dr. Bak's creativity. This time, they will stand in to ask the right questions to unleash that creative power in ways for others to follow the trail. Part of the MILLION DOLLAR MINDSET series, HOW TO BOOST YOUR CREATIVITY TO NEW HEIGHTS is Dr. Bak's open book to one of his superpowers.

In HOW TO NOT FAIL AS A DENTIST, Dr. Bak is given 20 plus years of experience and knowledge of what it is to be a dentist on the ground. PROFESSIONAL INTELLIGENCE, FINANCIAL INTELLIGENCE and MANAGEMENT INTELLIGENCE are the fields that any dentist will have to master for a chance to succeed and a shot at happiness, practicing dentistry. Where ever you are starting your career as a new graduate or a veteran in the field looking to reach the next level, this is book smart and street smart all into one. This is Million Dollar Mindset applied to dentistry. We won't be making a millionaire out of you from this book, we will be giving you a shot at happiness and success. The million will follow soon enough.

HOW TO WRITE A BOOK IN 30 DAYS -042

BY Dr. BAK NGUYEN

In HOW TO WRITE A BOOK IN 30 DAYS, after more than 100 books written in 4 years, Dr. Bak is revisiting his first hit, the book in which he shared his craft and structure of how to write books. After 100 books, Dr. Bak proved that not only content is important, but what will keep the words coming are the structure and the process. If you are looking into writing your first book, this is your chance. If you are thinking about it, do it, and as fast as possible. Writing your first book will set you free from your past and open the doors to your own future! Everyone has a story worth telling! Where to start, how to get by the INSPIRATIONAL WALL, what are the techniques to bring depth into your storytelling, how to structure your chapter, how many chapters, how to have a book, in a month? These are the answers you will find within HOW TO WRITE A BOOK IN 30 DAYS. You will find a wealth of wisdom from his experience writing your first, second or even 10th book. Dr. Bak is sharing his secrets writing books. By the way, he wrote this book and got it published within 6 days. Welcome to the Alphas.

HOW 2 WRITE 2 BOOKS IN 10 DAYS -114

BY WILLIAM & Dr. BAK NGUYEN

HOW 2 WRITE 2 BOOKS IN 10 DAYS, is William Bak takes on his father's hit, HOW TO WRITE A BOOK IN 30 DAYS. This time, William is covering the art of writing fiction. As mentioned in the title, William is writing this book and the next one within 10 days. Just not to mislead you, writing fiction will take longer, but once you have done all your prep work and research, it can be written as quickly. William is only 12 and already, he has signed 35 books. Most of his books are fiction, so on the matter, he is a veteran author, one with much experience of the ups and downs when it comes to writing books and getting them to the finish line Joining him is Dr. Bak who is sharing his secrets of writing fiction too. What does it take, how different it is from writing non-fictional books and what does it take to inspire and motivate his 12-year-old son to write as much, matching his world record pace? HOW 2 WRITE 2 BOOKS IN 10 DAYS is a joke between 2 world record authors teasing one another as they keep raising the bar higher and higher. Welcome to the Alphas.

HOW TO WRITE A SUCCESSFUL BUSINESS PLAN -049

BY Dr. BAK NGUYEN & ROUBA SAKR

In HOW TO WRITE A SUCCESSFUL BUSINESS PLAN, Dr. Bak is given 20 plus years of experience and knowledge of what it is to be an entrepreneur and more importantly, how to have the investors and banks on your side. Being an entrepreneur is surely not something you learn from school, but there are steps to master so you can communicate your views and vision. That's the only way you will have financing. Writing a business is only not a mandatory stop only for the bankers, but an essential step for every entrepreneur, to know the direction and what's coming next. A business plan is also not set in stone, if there is a truth in business is that nothing will go as planned. Writing down your business plan the first time will prepare you to adapt and overcome the challenges and surprises. For most entrepreneurs, a business is a passion. To most investors and all banks, a business is a system. Your business plan is the map to that system. However unique your ideas and business are, the mapping follows the same steps and pattern.

HOW TO SEDUCE ANYONE -129
BY Dr. BAK NGUYEN

In HOW TO SEDUCE ANYONE, Dr. Bak is pushed by 2 of his female apprentices to share the secret behind his smile and influence. Seduction has many facets and can be leveraged in so many ways. Dr. Bak's way is to seduce without seducing, with tricks or fireworks. He, himself never saw himself as a seducer, until asked to share his skills and knowledge on the matter. Everything in life is about connecting and interacting with others. So it is safe to say that all of our social life is about seducing, even when sharing. To learn to eat, to talk, to wrap, and to open is an old Vietnamese saying about the ways of life. Well, to Dr. Bak, it is much simpler than that. Seduction is about being confident enough to be available to the other person, available to listen and to empower. It is all about what the other person feels in your presence which is the key to your influence and charm. Easier said than done! Well in this journey, you are following Dr. Bak along with Alpha Coach Mel and Alpha host Natasha DG to uncover the ways to seduce without seducing, to gain the minds and hearts of those you touch without compromising or overselling yourself. HOW TO SEDUCE ANYONE is a conversation with Dr. Bak, straight from the heart and without filtre. Based on a podcast interview from WOMAN UP and more than 3 decades of winning the hearts of those he touches, these are Dr. Bak's secrets. Welcome to the Alphas.

HUMILITY FOR SUCCESS -051
BALANCING STRATEGY AND EMOTIONS
BY Dr. BAK NGUYEN

HUMILITY FOR SUCCESS is exploring the emotional discomforts and challenges champions, and overachievers put themselves through. Success is never done overnight and on the way, just like the pain and the struggles aren't enough, we are dealing with the doubts, the haters, and those who like to tell us how to live our lives and what to do. At the same time, nothing of worth can be achieved alone. Every legend has a cast of characters, allies, mentors, companions, rivals, and foes. So one needs the key to social behaviour. HUMILITY FOR SUCCESS is exploring the matter and will help you sort out beliefs from values, and peers from friends. Humility is much more about how we see ourselves than how others see us. For any entrepreneur and champion, our daily is to set our mindset right, and to perfect our skills, not to fit in. There is a world where CONFIDENCE grows in synergy with HUMILITY. As you set the right label on the right belief, you will be able to grow and leave the lies and haters far behind. This is HUMILITY FOR SUCCESS.

HYBRID -011
THE MODERN QUEST OF IDENTITY
BY Dr. BAK NGUYEN

IDENTITY -004
THE ANTHOLOGY OF QUESTS
BY Dr. BAK NGUYEN

What if John Lennon was still alive and running for president today? What kind of campaign will he be running? IDENTIFY -THE ANTHOLOGY OF QUESTS is about the quest each of us has to undertake, sooner or later, THE QUEST OF IDENTITY. Citizens of the world, aim to be one, the one, one whole, one unity, made of many. That's the anthology of life! Start with your one, find your unity, and your legend will start. We are all small-minded people anyway! We need each other to be one! We need each other to be happy, so we, so you, so I, can be happy. This is the chorus of life. This is our song! Citizens of the world, I salute you! This is the first tome of the IDENTITY QUEST. FORCES OF NATURE (tome 2) will be following in SUMMER 2021. Also under development, Tome 3 - THE CONQUEROR WITHIN will start production soon.

INDUSTRIES DISRUPTORS -006
BY Dr. BAK NGUYEN

INDUSTRIES DISRUPTORS is a strange title, one that sparkles mixed feelings. A disruptor is someone making a difference, and since we, in general, do not like change, the label is mostly negative. But a disruptor is mostly someone who sees the same problem and challenge from another angle. The disruptor will tackle that angle and come up with something new from something existent. That's evolution! In INDUSTRIES DISRUPTORS, Dr. Bak is joining forces with James Stephan-Usypchuk to share with us what is going on in the minds and shoes of those entrepreneurs disrupting the old habits. Dr. Bak is changing the world from a dental chair, disrupting the dental, and now the book industry. James is a maverick in the Intelligence space, from marketing to Artificial Intelligence. Coming from very different backgrounds and industries, they end up telling very similar stories. If disruptors change the world, well, their story proves that disruptors can be made and forged. Here's the recipe. Here are their stories.

K

KRYPTO -040
TO SAVE THE WORLD
BY Dr. BAK NGUYEN & ILYAS BAKOUCH

L

L'ART DE TRANSFORMER DE LA SOUPE EN MAGIE -103
PAR Dr. BAK NGUYEN

Dans L'ART DE TRANSFORMER DE LA SOUPE EN MAGIE, Dr. Bak remonte aux sources pour connaître la source de son génie et la recette qui a été transféré à son fils, William Bak, auteur et record mondial dès l'âge de 8 ans. Docteur en médecine dentaire, entrepreneur, écrivain record mondial, musicien, Dr. Bak est d'abord et avant tout un fils qui a une maman qui croit en lui. L'ART DE TRANSFORMER DE LA SOUPE EN MAGIE est dédié à la recette du génie, celle qui pousse une mère a mijoté les ingrédients de l'espoir dans un bouillon d'amour, à y ajuster un zeste de bonheur et un brin d'ambition. Dans la lignée des livres parentaux de Dr. Bak, L'ART DE TRANSFORMER DE LA SOUPE EN MAGIE est dédié à la première femme dans sa vie, celle qui a tracé son destin et celle qui l'a cultivée.

LEADERSHIP -003
PANDORA'S BOX
BY Dr. BAK NGUYEN

LEADERSHIP, PANDORA'S BOX is 21 presidential speeches for a better tomorrow for all of us. It aims to drive HOPE and motivation into each and every one of us. Together we can make the difference, we hold such power. Covering themes from LOYALTY to GENEROSITY, from FREEDOM and INTELLIGENCE to DOUBTS and DEATH, this is not the typical presidential or motivational speeches that we are used to. LEADERSHIP PANDORA'S BOX will surf your emotions first, only to dive with you to touch the core and soul of our meaning: to matter. This is not a Quest of Identity, but the cry to rally as a species, raise our heads toward the future and move forward as a WHOLE. Not a typical Dr. Bak's book, LEADERSHIP, PANDORA'S BOX is a must-read for all of you looking for hope and purpose, all of us, citizens of the world.

LEADERSHIP vol. 1 (ALPHA DENTISTRY) -121
CHANGING THE WORLD FROM A DENTAL CHAIR

🏴 ALBANIA 🇧🇷 BRAZIL 🇨🇦 CANADA 🏳 HUNGARY 🇲🇾 MALAYSIA 🏴 SPAIN 🇺🇸 USA
BY Dr. BAK NGUYEN, Dr. MAHSA KHAGHANI, Dr. NAGY KATALIN, with guest authors Dr. PAUL DOMINIQUE, Dr. PAUL OUELLETTE, Dr. GURIEN DEMIRAQI, Dr. BENNETE FERNANDES, Dr. SANDRA FABIANO, Dr. ARASH HAKHAMIAN and Dr. MARILYN SANDOR

ALPHA DENTISTRY proudly presents LEADERSHIP, CHANGING THE WORLD FROM A DENTAL CHAIR. This time, Dr. Bak is leading the charge of rebuilding the foundations of the dental industry, especially after the light shed by COVID. More than once, populations from all around the world have expressed their negative perceptions and uneasy feelings about the dental industry. For decades, we turned deaf and blinded to these criticisms. In the worse health crisis of our lifetime, our specialists, experts and all our doctors were benched, despite being health professionals... The message is clear, the whole field must be rethought and better adapted to our modern societies. In the hope of bringing new ideas and philosophies, Dr. Bak is joined by Dr. Mahsa Khaghani from Spain and Dr. Nagy Katalin from Hungary, along with Dr. Paul Dominique, Dr. Paul Ouellette, Dr. Arash Hakhamian and Dr. Marilyn Sandor from the USA, Dr. Gurien Demiraqi from Albania, Dr. Bennete Fernandes from Malaysia, and Dr. Sandra Fabiano from Brazil to lead this history journey looking to modernize and make dentistry more accessible and affordable. It will take leadership and courage to assemble all of the world's dental industry and bridge the gaps to a better future. It starts by listening and then, dialoguing. LEADERSHIP is an inclusive dialogue. This is the first volume of this new series in which International Dental leaders will be joining forces to rebuild Dentistry. First mission: lower the costs of dentistry. Welcome to the Alphas.

LEGENDS OF DESTINY vol.1 -101
THE PROLOGUES OF DESTINY

BY Dr. BAK NGUYEN & WILLIAM BAK

The war between the forces of death and the legions of life lasted for centuries, ravaging most of the twin planets, Destiny and Earth. The end was so imminent that even the Gods got involved to save Life from eternal doom. Heroes rise and fall from all sides. Some fight for good, others, for evil. Gods, titans, angels, and demons all took sides in the war. Gods fight and kill other gods. Angel fights alongside demons, striking down Gods and Titans, and rival angels. The war lasted for so long that no one even remembers what they were fighting for. Some fight for domination while others, just to survive. The war ravages Destiny, the twin sister of planet Earth to the brink of annihilation. All eyes now turn to Earth. As the balance of the creation itself hands in the balance, a species emerges as holding the balance to victory: mankind. For the future of Humanity, of Gods and men and everything in between, this is the last stand of Destiny, a last chance for life.

LEGENDS OF DESTINY vol.2 -107
THE BOOK OF ELVES

BY Dr. BAK NGUYEN & WILLIAM BAK

Caught between the Orcs invading from the center of Destiny, the Angels raining down and the Demons eating from within, the Elves are turning from their old beliefs and Gods for salvation. For Millennials, Elves turned to Odin and the Forces of Nature for answers and guidance. Since the imminent destruction of their kingdoms and cities, a new God is offering Hope, Kal, the old God of fire. Kal gave them more than Hope, he gave the elves who turned to him for passage to a new world. But more than hope, more than fear, Elves value honour and Destiny. At least their old guards and heroes do. With their world crumbling down, and the rise of the new and younger generations, Elf's society seems to be at the crossroad of evolution. It is convert or die. Or die fighting or die kneeling. The Book of Elves is the story of a civilization facing its fate in the blink of destruction.

LE POUVOIR DE LA SÉDUCTION -130

PAR Dr. BAK NGUYEN

Dans LE POUVOIR DE LA SÉDUCTION, le Dr Bak est poussé par deux de ses protégées Alphas à partager le secret derrière son sourire et son influence. La séduction a de nombreuses facettes et peut être utilisée à de nombreuses fins. Séduire sans séduire, est la philosophie du Dr. Bak, sans astuces ni feux d'artifice. Lui-même ne s'est jamais considéré comme un séducteur jusqu'à ce qu'on le sollicite pour ses compétences et secrets en la matière. La vie sociale est une grande séduction. Que ce soit d'interagir, partager, soigner, enseigner, même aider, tout revient sur l'aptitude de chacun à mettre en confiance. Apprendre à manger, à parler, à emballer et à ouvrir est un vieux dicton vietnamien sur la façon de vivre. Eh bien, pour le Dr Bak, c'est beaucoup plus simple que cela. La séduction consiste à être suffisamment confiant pour pouvoir s'oublier et être disponible pour l'autre.

La clé de la séduction et de l'influence est dans comment les autres se sentent en notre présence. LE POUVOIR DE LA SÉDUCTION est une conversation entre avec la coach Mel et l'animatrice Natasha DG, le Dr Bak et vous. Ce livre est inspiré du podcast WOMAN UP et sur plus de 3 décennies à conquérir les cœurs et le respect de ceux qu'il touche. Voici les secrets du Dr Bak. Bienvenu(e) aux Alphas.

LEVERAGE -014
COMMUNICATION INTO SUCCESS
BY Dr. BAK NGUYEN

In LEVERAGE COMMUNICATION TO SUCCESS, Dr. Bak shares his secret and mindsets to elevate an idea into a vision and a vision into an endeavour. Some endeavours will be a project, some others will become companies, and some will grow into a movement. It does not matter, each started with great communication. Communication is a very vast concept, education, sale, sharing, empowering, coaching, preaching, and entertaining. Those are all different kinds of communication. The intent differs, the audiences vary, and the messages are unique but the frame can be templated and mastered. In LEVERAGE COMMUNICATION TO SUCCESS, Dr. Bak is loyal to his core, sharing only what he knows best, what he has done himself. This book is dedicated to communicating successfully in business.

M

MASTERMIND, 7 WAYS INTO THE BIG LEAGUE -052
BY Dr. BAK NGUYEN & JONAS DIOP

MASTERMIND, 7 WAYS INTO THE BIG LEAGUE is the result of the encounter between business coach Jonas Diop and Dr. Bak. As a professional podcaster and someone always seeking the truth and ways to leverage success and performance, coach Jonas is putting Dr. Bak to the test, one that should reveal his secret to overachieve month after month, accumulating a new world record every month. Follow those two great minds as they push each other to surpass themselves, each in their own way and own style. MASTERMIND, 7 WAYS INTO THE BIG LEAGUE is more than a roadmap to success, it is a journey and a live testimony as you are turning the pages, one by one.

MENTORSHIP 133
BY Dr. BAK NGUYEN & COACH MEL

MENTORSHIP, THE POWER OF SHARING is the conversation between a mentor and his apprentice. This is a journey of discovery, of healing, and of empowerment. Power and wisdom don't fade with time, they morph stronger and shapeless if one can renew purpose. Walking legends, writing history, even for seduction, one needs to understand and master the POWER OF MIRRORS to grow, to win. The power of mirrors is the only power that won't corrupt its host. It might blind, but not corrupt. And the only way to avoid blindness in the light of great power is to have a mirror to react to. This is the essence of a mentor/apprentice relationship. To the apprentice, it is the privilege to gain much power and wisdom. To the mentor, it is the chance to break the limits of his or her own power to ascend into even greater power. MENTORSHIP, THE POWER OF SHARING is the conversation between Dr. Bak and Coach Mel, on her path to setting the next world record mark in literature, beating her mentor. It is the universal dynamic of every mentor-apprentice synergy. Welcome to the Alphas.

MIDAS TOUCH 065
POST-COVID DENTISTRY
BY Dr. BAK NGUYEN, Dr. JULIO REYNAFARJE AND Dr. PAUL OUELLETTE

MIDAS TOUCH, is the memoir of what happened in the ALPHAS SUMMIT in the midst of the GREAT PAUSE as great minds throughout the world in the dental field are coming together. As the time of competition is obsolete, the new era of collaboration is blooming. This is the 3rd book of the ALPHAS, after AFTERMATH and RELEVANCY, all written in the midst of confinement. Dr. Julio Reynafarje is bearing this initiative, to share with you the secret of a successful and lasting relationship with your patients, balancing science and psychology, kindness, and professionalism. He personally invited the ALPHAS to join as co-author, Dr. Paul Ouellette, Dr. Paul Dominique, and Dr. Bak. Together, they have more than 100 years of combined experience, wisdom, trade, skills, philosophy, and secrets to share with you to empower you in the rebuilding of the dental profession in the aftermath of COVID. RELEVANCY was about coming together and rebuilding the future. MIDAS TOUCH is about how to build, one treatment plan at a time, one story at a time, one smile at a time.

MINDSET ARMORY -050

BY Dr. BAK NGUYEN

MINDSET ARMORY is Dr. Bak's 49th book, days after he completed his world record of writing 48 books within 24 months, on top of being the CEO of Mdex & Co and a full-time cosmetic dentist. Dr. Bak is undoubtedly an OVERACHIEVER. In his last books, he has shared more and more of his lifestyle and how it forged his winning mindset. Within MINDSET ARMORY, Dr. Bak is sharing with us his tools, how he found them, forged them, and leverage them. Just like any warrior needs a shield, a sword, and a ride, here are Dr. Bak's. For any entrepreneur, the road to success is a long and winding journey. On the way, some will find allies and foes. Some allies will become foes, and some foes might become allies. In today's competitive world, the only constant is change. With the right tool, it is possible to achieve. The right tool, the right mindset. This is MINDSET ARMORY.

MIRROR -085

BY Dr. BAK NGUYEN

MIRROR is the theme for a personal book. Not only to Dr. Bak but to all of us looking to reach beyond who and what we actually are. MIRROR is special in the fact that it is not only the content of the book that is of worth but the process in which Dr. Bak shared his own evolution. To go beyond who we are, one must grow every day. And how do you compare your growth and how far have you reached? Looking in the mirror. In all of Dr. Bak's writing, looking at the past is a trap to avoid at all costs. Looking in the mirror, is that any better? Share Dr. Bak's way to push and keep pushing himself without friction or resistance. Please read that again. To evolve without friction or resistance... that is the source of infinite growth and the unification of the Quest for Power and the Quest of Happiness.

MOMENTUM TRANSFER -009

BY Dr. BAK NGUYEN & Coach DINO MASSON

How to be successful in your business and life? Achieve Your Biggest Goals With MOMENTUM TRANSFER. START THE BUSINESS YOU WANT - AND BRING IT NEXT LEVEL! GET THE LIFE YOU ALWAYS WANTED - AND IMPROVE IT! TAKE ANY PROJECTS YOU HAVE - AND MAKE THEM THE BEST! In this powerful book, you'll discover what a small business owner learnt from a millionaire and successful entrepreneur. He applied his mentor's principles and is explaining them in full detail in this book. The small business owner wrote the book he has always wanted to read and went from the verge of bankruptcy to quadrupling his revenues in less than 9 months and improve his personal life by increasing his energy and bringing back peacefulness. Together, the millionaire and the small business owner are sharing their most valuable business and life lessons with the world. The most powerful book to increase your momentum in your business and your life introduces simple and radical life-changing concepts: Multiply your business revenues by finding the Eye of your Momentum - Increase your energy by building and feeding your own Momentum - How to increase your confidence with these simple steps - How to transfer your new powerful energy into other aspects of your business and life - How to set goals and achieve them (even crush them!)- How to always tap into an effortless and limitless force within you- And much, much more!

P

PLAYBOOK INTRODUCTION -055
BY Dr. BAK NGUYEN

In PLAYBOOK INTRODUCTION, Dr. Bak is open the door to all the newcomers and aspirant entrepreneurs who are looking at where and when to start. Based on questions of two college students wanting to know how to start their entrepreneurial journey, Dr. Bak dives into his experiences to empower the next generation, not about what they should do, but how he, Dr. Bak, would have done it today. This is an important aspect to recognize in the business world, the world has changed since the INFORMATION AGE and the advent of the millenniums into the market. Most matrix and know-how have to be adapted to today's speed and accessibility to the information. We are living at the INFORMATION AGE, this book is the precursor to the ABUNDANCE AGE, at least to those open to embracing the opportunity.

PLAYBOOK INTRODUCTION 2 -056
BY Dr. BAK NGUYEN

In PLAYBOOK INTRODUCTION 2, Dr. Bak continues the journey to welcome the newcomers and aspirant entrepreneurs looking at where and when to start. If the first volume covers the mindset, the second is covering much more in-depth the concept of debt and leverage. This is an important aspect to recognize in the business world, the world has changed since the INFORMATION AGE and the advent of the millenniums into the market. Most matrix and know-how have to be adapted to today's speed and accessibility to the information. We are living at the INFORMATION AGE, this book is the precursor to the ABUNDANCE AGE, at least to those open to embrace the opportunity.

POWER -043
EMOTIONAL INTELLIGENCE
BY Dr. BAK NGUYEN

IN POWER, EMOTIONAL INTELLIGENCE, Dr. Bak is sharing his experiences and secrets leveraging on his EMOTIONAL INTELLIGENCE, a power we all have within. From SYMPATHY, having others opening up to you, to ACTIVE LISTENING, saving you time and energy; from EMPATHY, allowing you to predict the future to INFLUENCE, enabling you to draft the future, not to forget the power of the crowd with MOMENTUM, you are now in possession of power in tune with nature, yourself. It is a unique take on the subject to empower you to find your powers and your destiny. Visionary businessman, and doctor in dentistry, Dr. Bak describes himself as a Dentist by circumstances, a communicator by passion, and an entrepreneur by nature.

POWERPLAY -078
HOW TO BUILD THE PERFECT TEAM
BY Dr. BAK NGUYEN

In POWERPLAY, HOW TO BUILD THE PERFECT TEAM, Dr. Bak is sharing with you his experience, perspective, and mistake travelling the journey of the entrepreneur. A serial entrepreneur himself, he started venture only with a single partner as a team to build companies with a director of human resources and a board of directors. POWERPLAY is not a story, it is the HOW TO build the perfect team, knowing that perfection is a lie. So how can one build a team that will empower his or her vision? How to recruit, how to train, how to retain? Those are all legitimate questions. And all of those won't matter if the first question isn't answered: what is the reason for the team? There is the old way to hire and the new way to recruit. Yes, Human Resources is all about mindset too! This journey is one of introspection, of leadership, and a cheat sheet to build, not only the perfect team but the team that will empower your legacy to the next level.

PROFESSION HEALTH - TOME ONE -005
THE UNCONVENTIONAL QUEST OF HAPPINESS
BY Dr. BAK NGUYEN, Dr. MIRJANA SINDOLIC, Dr. ROBERT DURAND AND COLLABORATORS

Why are health professionals burning out while they give the best of themselves to heal the world? Dr. Bak aims to break the curse of isolation that health professionals face and establish a conversation to start the healing process. PROFESSION HEALTH is the basis of an ongoing discussion and will also serve as an introduction to a study led by Professor Robert Durand, DMD, MSc Science from the University of Montreal, a study co-financed by Mdex and the Federal Government of Canada. Co-writers are Dr. Mirjana Sindolic, Professor Robert Durand, Dr. Jean De Serres, MD and former President of Hema Quebec, Counsel-Minister Luis Maria Kalaff Sanchez, Dr. Miguel Angel Russo, MD, Banker Anthony Siggia, Banker Kyles Yves, and more… This is the first Tome of three, dedicated to helping "WHITE COATS" to heal and to find their happiness.

R

REBOOT -012
MIDLIFE CRISIS
BY Dr. BAK NGUYEN

MidLife Crisis is a common theme for each of us as we reach the threshold. As a man, as a woman, why is it that half of the marriages end up in recall? If anything else would have half those rates of failure, the lawsuits would be raining. Where are the flaws, the traps?

Love is strong and pure, why is marriage not the reflection of that? Those are all hard questions to ask with little or no answers. Dr. Bak is sharing his reflections and findings as he reached himself the WALL OF MARRIAGE. This is a matter that affects all of our lives. It is time for some answers.

RELEVANCY - TOME TWO -064
REINVENTING OURSELVES TO SURVIVE
BY Dr. BAK NGUYEN & Dr. PAUL OUELLETTE AND COLLABORATORS

THE GREAT PAUSE was a reboot of all the systems of society. Many outdated systems will not make it back. The Dental Industry is a needed one, it has laid on complacency for far too long. In an age where expertise is global and democratized and can be replaced with technologies and artificial intelligence, the REBOOT will force, not just an update, but an operating system replacement and a firmware upgrade. First, they saved their industry with THE ALPHAS INITIATIVE, sharing their knowledge and vision freely to all the world's dental industry. With the OUELLETTE INITIATIVE, they bought some time for all the dental clinics to resume and adjust. The warning has been given, the clock is now ticking. who will prevail and prosper and who will be left behind, outdated and obsolete?

RISING -062
TO WIN MORE THAN YOU ARE AFRAID TO LOSE
BY Dr. BAK NGUYEN

In RISING, TO WIN MORE TAN YOU ARE AFRAID TO LOSE, Dr. Bak is breaking down the strategy to success to all, not only those wearing white coats and scrubs. More than his previous book (SUCCESS IS A CHOICE), this one is covering most of the aspects of getting to the next level, psychologically, socially, and financially. Rising is broken down into three key strategies: Financial Leverage - Compressing time - Always being in control. Presented by MILLION DOLLAR MINDSET, the book is covering more than the ways to create wealth, but also how to reach happiness and live a life without regrets. Dr. Bak the CEO and founder of Mdex & Co, a company with the promise of reforming the whole dental industry for the better. He wrote more than 60 books within 30 months as he is sharing his experiences, secrets, and wisdom.

S

SELFMADE -036
GRATITUDE AND HUMILITY
BY Dr. BAK NGUYEN

This is the story of Dr. Bak, an artist who became a dentist, a dentist who became an Entrepreneur, an Entrepreneur who is seeking to save an entire industry. In his free time, Dr. Bak managed to write 37 books and is a contender for 3 world records to be confirmed. Businessman and visionary, his views and philosophy are ahead of our time. This is his 37th book. In SELFMADE, Dr. Bak is answering the questions most entrepreneurs want to know, the HOWTO and the secret recipes, not just to succeed, but to keep going no matter what! SELFMADE is the perfect read for any entrepreneurs, novices, and veterans.

SHORTCUT vol. 1 - HEALING -093
BY Dr. BAK NGUYEN

In SHORTCUT 408 HEALING QUOTES, Dr. Bak revisits and compiles his journey of healing and growing. Just like anyone, he was moulded and shaped by Conformity and Society to the point of blending and melting. Walking his journey of healing, he rediscovers himself and found his true calling. And once whole with himself and with the Universe, Dr. Bak found his powers. In SHORTCUT 408 HEALING QUOTES, you have a quick and easy way to surf his mindsets and what allowed him to heal, to find back his voice and wings, and to walk his destiny. You too are walking your Quest of Identity. That one is mainly a journey of healing. May you find yours and your powers.

SHORTCUT vol. 2 - GROWING -094
BY Dr. BAK NGUYEN

In SHORTCUT 408 GROWTH QUOTES, Dr. Bak is compiling his library of books about personal growth and self-improvement. More than a motivational book, more than a compilation of knowledge, Dr. Bak is sharing the mindsets upon which he found his power to achieve and to overachieve. We all have our powers, only they were muted and forgotten as we were forged by Conformity and Society. After the healing process, walking your Quest of Identity, the Quest for your growth and God-given power is next to lead you to walk your Destiny.

SHORTCUT vol. 3 - LEADERSHIP -095
BY Dr. BAK NGUYEN

In SHORTCUT 365 LEADERSHIP QUOTES, Dr. Bak is compiling his library of books about leadership and ambition. Yes, the ambition is to find your worth and to make the world a better place for all of us. If the 3rd volume of SHORTCUT is mainly a motivational compilation, it also holds the secrets and mindsets to influence and leadership. If you were looking to walk your legend and impact the world, you are walking a lonely path. You might on your own, but it does not have to be harder than it is. As we all have your unique challenges, the key to victory is often found in the same place, your heart. And here are 365 shortcuts to keep you believing and to attract more people to you as you are growing into a true leader.

SHORTCUT vol. 4 - CONFIDENCE 096
BY Dr. BAK NGUYEN

SHORTCUT 518 CONFIDENCE QUOTES, is the most voluminous compilation of Dr. Bak's quotes. To heal was the first step. To grow and find your powers came next. As you are walking your personal legend, Confidence is both your sword and armour to conquer your Destiny and overcome all of the challenges on your way. In SHORTCUT volume four, Dr. Bak comprises all his mindsets and wisdom to ease your ascension. Confidence is not something one is simply born with, but something to nurture, grow, and master. Some will have the chance to be raised by people empowering Confidence, others will have to heal from Conformity to grow their confidence. It does not matter, only once Confident, can one stand tall and see clearly the horizon.

SHORTCUT vol. 5- SUCCESS -097
BY Dr. BAK NGUYEN

Success is not a destination but a journey and a side effect. While no map can lead you to success, the right mindset will forge your own success, the one without medals nor labels. If you are looking to walk your legend, to be successful is merely the beginning. Actually, being successful is often a side effect of the mindsets and actions that you took, you provoked. In SHORTCUT 317 SUCCESS QUOTES, Dr. Bak is revisiting his journey, breaking down what led him to be successful despite the odds stacked against him. As success is the consequence of mindsets, choices, and actions, it can be duplicated over and over again, one just needs to master the mindsets first.

SHORTCUT vol. 6- POWER -098
BY Dr. BAK NGUYEN

That's the kind of power that you will discover within this journey. Power is a tool, a leverage. Well used, it will lead to great achievements. Misused, it will be your downfall. If a sword sometimes has 2 edges, Power is a sword with no handle and multiple edges. You have been warned. In SHORTCUT 376 POWER QUOTES, Dr. Bak is compiling all the powers he found and mastered walking his own legend. If the first power was Confidence, very quickly, Dr. Bak realized that Confidence was the key to many, many more powers. Where to find them, how to yield them, and how to leverage these powers is the essence of the 6th volume of SHORTCUT.

SHORTCUT vol. 7- HAPPINESS -099
BY Dr. BAK NGUYEN

We were all born happy and then, somehow, we lost our ways and forgot our ways home. Is this the real tragedy behind the lost paradise myth? If we were happy once, we can trust our hearts to find our way home, once more. This is the journey of the 7th volume of the SHORTCUT series. In SHORTCUT 306 HAPPINESS QUOTES, Dr. Bak is revisiting and compiling all the secrets and mindsets leading to happiness. Happiness is not just a destination but a shrine for Confidence and a safe place to regroup, to heal, to grow. We each have our own happiness. What you will learn here is where to find yours and, more importantly, how to leverage you to ease the journey ahead, because happiness is not your final destination. It can be the key to your legend.

SHORTCUT vol. 8- DOCTORS -100
BY Dr. BAK NGUYEN

If healing was the first step to your destiny and powers, there is a science to healing. Those with that science are doctors, the healers of the world. In India, healers are second only to the Gods! In SHORTCUT 170 DOCTOR QUOTES, Dr. Bak is dedicating the 8th volume of the series to his peers, doctors, from all around the world. Doctors too, have to walk their Quest of Identity, to heal from their pain and to walk their legend. Doctors need to heal and rejuvenate to keep healing the world. If healing is their science, in SHORTCUT, they will access the power of leveraging.

SUCCESS IS A CHOICE -060
BLUEPRINTS FOR HEALTH PROFESSIONALS
BY Dr. BAK NGUYEN

In SUCCESS IS A CHOICE, FINANCIAL MILLIONAIRE BLUEPRINTS FOR HEALTH PROFESSIONALS, Dr. Bak is breaking down the strategy to success for all those wearing white coats and scrubs: doctors, dentists, pharmacists, chiropractors, nurses, etc. Success is broken down into three key strategies: Financial Leverage - Compressing time - Always being in control. Presented by MILLION DOLLAR MINDSET, the book is covering more than the ways to create wealth, but also how to reach happiness and live a life without regrets. Dr. Bak is a successful cosmetic dentist with nearly 20 years of experience. He founded Mdex & Co, a company with the promise of reforming the whole dental industry for the better. While doing so, he discovered a passion for writing and for sharing. Multiple times World Record, Dr. Bak is writing a book every 2 weeks for the last 30 months. This is his 60th book, and he is still practicing. How he does it, is what he is sharing with us, SUCCESS, HAPPINESS, and mostly FREEDOM to all Health Professionals.

SYMPHONY OF SKILLS -001
BY Dr. BAK NGUYEN

You will enlighten the world with your potential. I can't wait to see all the differences that you will have in our world. Remember that power comes with responsibility. We can feel in his presence, a genuine force, a depth of energy, confidence, innocence, courage, and intelligence. Bak is always looking for answers, morning and night, he wants to understand the why and the why not. This book is the essence of the man. Dr. Bak is a force of nature who bears proudly his title eHappy. The man never ceases smiling and spreading his good vibe wherever he passes. He is not trapped in the nostalgia of the past nor the satisfaction of the present, he embodies the joy of what's possible, and what's to come. The more we read, the more we share, and we live. That is Bak, he charms us to evolve and to share his points of view, and before we know it, we are walking by his side, a journey we never saw coming.

T

THE 90 DAYS CHALLENGE -061
BY Dr. BAK NGUYEN

THE 90 DAYS CHALLENGE, is Dr. Bak's journey into the unknown. Overachiever writing 2 books a month on average, for the last 30 months, ambitious CEO, Industries' Disruptor, Dr. Bak seems to have success in everything he touches. Everything except the control of his weight. For nearly 20 years, he struggles with an overweight problem. Every time he scored big, he added on a little more weight. Well, this time, he exposes himself out there, in real-time and without filter, accepting the challenge of his brother-in-law, DON VO to lose 45 pounds within 90 days. That's half a pound a day, for three months. He will have to do so while keeping all of his other challenges on track, writing books at a world record pace, leading the dental industry into the new ERA, and keep seeing his patients. Undoubtedly entertaining, this is the journey of an ALPHA who simply won't give up. But this time, nothing is sure.

THE BOOK OF LEGENDS -024
BY Dr. BAK NGUYEN & WILLIAM BAK

The Book of Legends vol. 1 is the story behind the world record of Dr. Bak and his son, William Bak. All Dr. Bak had in mind was to keep his promise of writing a book with his son. They ended up writing 8 children's books within a month, scoring a new world record.

William is also the youngest author having published in two languages. Those are world records waiting to be confirmed. History will say: to celebrate a first world record (writing 15 books / 15 months), for the love of his son, he will have scored a second world record: to write 8 books within a month! THE BOOK OF LEGENDS vol. 1 This is both a magical journey for both a father and a son looking to connect and find themselves. Join Dr. Bak and William Bak in their journey and their love for Life!

THE BOOK OF LEGENDS 2 -041
BY Dr. BAK NGUYEN & WILLIAM BAK

THE BOOK OF LEGENDS vol. 2 is the sequel of "CINDERELLA" but a true story between a father and his son. Together they have discovered a bond and a way to connect. The first BOOK OF LEGENDS covered the time of the first four books they wrote together within a month. The second BOOK OF LEGENDS is covering what happened after the curtains dropped, and what happened after reality kicked back in. If the first volume was about a fairy tale in vacation time, the second volume is about making it last in real Life. Share their journey and their love of Life!

THE BOOK OF LEGENDS 3 -086
THE END OF THE INNOCENCE AGE
BY Dr. BAK NGUYEN & WILLIAM BAK

THE BOOK OF LEGENDS 3 is a long work extending to almost 3 years. If the shocking duo known as Dr. Bak and prodigy William Bak has marked the imaginary writing world record upon world record, the story is not all pink. After the franchise of the CHICKEN BOOKS, William, now in his pre-teen years, wants to move away from the chicken tales. After 22 chicken books, a break is well deserved. that said, what is next? Both father and son thought that if they could do it once easily, they could do it again! They couldn't be any further from the truth. For 2 years, they were stuck in the quest for their next franchise of books. THE BOOK OF LEGENDS 3 started right around the end of the chicken franchise and would have ended with a failure if the book was to be released on time, the holiday season of that year. It took the duo another year to complete their story to add the last chapters of this book, hoping to end with a happy ending. Unfortunately, not all story ends the way we wish… this is the dark tome of the series, where the imagination got eclipsed. Follow William and Dr. Bak in their fight to keep the magic and connection alive.

THE CONFESSION OF A LAZY OVERACHIEVER -089
REINVENT YOURSELF FROM ANY CRISIS
BY Dr. BAK NGUYEN

In THE CONFESSION OF A LAZY OVERACHIEVER, Dr. Bak is opening up to his new marketing officer, Jamie, fresh out of school. She is young, full of energy, and looking to chill and still have it all. True to his character, Dr. Bak is giving Jamie some leeway to redefine Dr. Bak's brand to her demographic, the Millennials. This journey is about Dr. Bak satisfying the Millennials and answering their true questions in life. A rebel himself, his ambition to change the world started back on campus, some 25 years ago... then, life caught up with him. It took Dr. Bak 20 years to shake down the burdens of life, spread his wings free from Conformity, and start Overachieving. Doctor, CEO, and world record author, here is what Dr. Bak would have loved to know 25 years ago as was still on campus. In a word, this is cheating your way to success and freedom. And yes, it is possible. Success, Money, and Freedom, they all start with a mindset and the awareness of Time. Welcome to the Alphas.

THE ENERGY FORMULA -053
BY Dr. BAK NGUYEN

THE ENERGY FORMULA is a book dedicated to helping each individual to find the means to reach their purpose and goal in Life. Dr. Bak is a philosopher, a strategist, a business, an artist, and a dentist, how does he do all of that? He is doing so while mentoring proteges and leading the modernization of an entire industry. Until now, Momentum and Speed were the powers that he was building on and from. But those powers come from somewhere too. From a guide of our Quest of Identity, he became an ally in everyone's journey for happiness. THE ENERGY FORMULA is the book revealing step by step, the logic of building the right mindset and the way to ABUNDANCE and HAPPINESS, universally. It is not just a HOW TO book, but one that will change your life and guide you to the path of ABUNDANCE.

THE MODERN WOMAN -070
TO HAVE IT HAVE WITH NO SACRIFICE
BY Dr. BAK NGUYEN & Dr. EMILY LETRAN

In THE MODERN WOMAN: TO HAVE IT ALL WITH NO SACRIFICE, Dr. Bak joins forces with Dr. Emily Letran to empower all women to fulfill their desires, goals, and ambition. Both overachievers going against the odds, they are sharing their experience and wisdom to help all women to find confidence and support to redefine their lives. Dr. Emily Letran is a doctor in dentistry, an entrepreneur, author, and CERTIFIED HIGH-PERFORMANCE coach. For an Asian woman, she made it through the norms and the red tapes to find her voice. As she learnt and grew with mentors, today she is sharing her secret with the energy that will motivate all of the female genders to stand for what they deserve. Alpha doctor, Bak is joining his voice and perspective since this is not about gender equality, but about personal empowerment and the quest of Identity of each, man and woman. Once more, Dr. Bak is bringing LEVERAGE and REASON to the new social deal between man and woman. This is not about gender, but about confidence.

THE POWER BEHIND THE ALPHA -008
BY TRANIE VO & Dr. BAK NGUYEN

It's been said by a "great man" that "We are born alone and we die alone." Both men and women proudly repeat those words as wisdom since. I apologize in advance, but what a fat LIE! That's what I learnt and discovered in life since my mind and heart got liberated from the burden of scars and the ladders of society. I can have it all, not all at the same time, but I can have everything I put my mind and heart into. Actually, it is not completely true. I can have most of what I and Tranie put our minds into. Together, when we feel like one, there isn't much out of our reach. If I'm the mind, she's the heart; if I'm the Will, she's the means. Synergy is the core of our power. Tranie's aim is always Happiness. In Tranie's definition of life, there are no justifications, no excuses, no tomorrow. For Tranie, Happiness is measured by the minutes of every single day. This is why she's so strong and can heal people around her. That may also be why she doesn't need to talk much, since talking about the past or the future is, in her mind, dimming down the magic of the present, the Now. We both respect and appreciate that we are the whole balancing each other's equation of life, of love, of success. I was the plus and the minus, then I became the multiplication factor and grew into the exponential. And how is Tranie evolving in all of this? She is and always will be the balance. If anything, she is the equal sign of each equation.

THE POWER OF Dr. -066
THE MODERN TITLE OF NOBILITY
BY Dr. BAK NGUYEN, Dr. PAVEL KRASTEV AND COLLABORATORS

In THE POWER OF Dr., independent thinkers mean to exchange ideas. An idea can be very powerful if supported by a great work ethic. Work ethic, isn't that the main fabric of our white coats, scrubs, and title? In an era post-COVID where everything has been rebooted and that's the healthcare industry is facing its own fate: to evolve or to be replaced, Dr. Bak and Dr. Pavel reveal the source of their power and their playbook to move forward, ahead.

The power we all hold is our resilience and discipline. We put that for years at the service of our profession, from a surgical perspective. Now, we can harness that same power to rewrite the rules, the industry, and our future. Post-COVID, the rules are being rewritten, will you be part of the team or left behind? "You can be in control!" More than personal growth and a motivational book, THE POWER OF Dr. is an awakening call to the doctor you look at when you graduate, with hope, with honour, with determination.

THE POWER OF YES -010
VOLUME ONE: IMPACT
BY Dr. BAK NGUYEN

In THE POWER OF YES, Dr. Bak is sharing his journey, opening up and embracing the world, one day at a time, one task at a time, one wish at a time. Far from a dare, saying YES allowed Dr. Bak to rewrite his mindset and break all the boundaries. This book is not one written in a few days or weeks, but the accumulation of a journey for 12 months. The journey started as Dr. Bak said YES to his producer to go on stage and speak... That YES opened a world of possibilities. Dr. Bak embraced each and every one of them. 12 months later, he is celebrating the new world record of writing 9 books written over a period of 12 months. To him, it will be a miss, missing the 12 on 12 mark. To the rest of the world, they just saw the birth of a force of nature, the Alpha force. THE POWER OF YES is comprised of all the introductions of the adult books written by Dr. Bak within the first 12 months. Chapter by chapter, you can walk in his footstep seeing and smelling what he has. This is reality-literature with a twist of POWER. THE POWER OF YES! Discover your potential and your power. This is the POWER OF YES, volume one. Welcome to the Alphas.

THE POWER OF YES 2 -037
VOLUME TWO: SHAPELESS
BY Dr. BAK NGUYEN

In THE POWER OF YES, volume 2, Dr. Bak is continuing his journey, discovering his powers and influence. After 12 months of embracing the world by saying YES, he rose as an emerging force: he's been recognized as an INDUSTRIES DISRUPTOR, got nominated ERNST AND YOUNG ENTREPRENEUR OF THE YEAR, wrote 9 books within 12 months while launching the most ambitious private endeavour to reform his own industry, the dental field. Contender too many WORLD RECORDS, Dr. Bak is doing all of that in parallel. And yes, he is sleeping his nights and yes, he is writing his book himself, from the screen of his iPhone! Far from satisfied, Dr. Bak missed the mark of writing 12 books within 12 months.

While everything is taking shape, everything could also crumble down at each turn. Now that Dr. Bak understands his powers, he is looking to test them and push them to their limits, looking to keep scoring world records while materializing his vision and enterprises. This is the awakening of a Force of Nature looking to change the world for the better while having fun sharing. Welcome to the Alphas.

THE POWER OF YES 3 -046
VOLUME THREE: LIMITLESS
BY Dr. BAK NGUYEN

In THE POWER OF YES, volume 3, the journey of Dr. Bak continues where the last volume left, in front of 300 plus people showing up to his first solo event, a Dr. Bak's event. On stage and in this book, Dr. Bak reveals how 12 months of saying YES to everything changed his life… actually, it was 18 months. From a dentist looking to change the world from a dental chair into a multiple times world record author, the journey of openness is a rendezvous with Fate. Dr. Bak is sharing almost in real-time his journey, and experiences, but above all, his feelings, doubts, and comebacks. From one book to the next, from one journey to the next, follow the adventure of a man looking to find his name, his worth, and his place in the world. Doing so, he is touching people Doing so, he is touching people and initiating their rise. Are you ready for more? Are you ready to meet your Fate and Destiny? Welcome to the Alphas.

THE POWER OF YES 4 -087
VOLUME FOUR: RISING
BY Dr. BAK NGUYEN

In THE POWER OF YES, volume 4, the journey continues days after where the last volume left. After setting the new world record of writing 48 books within 24 months, Dr. Bak is not ready to stop. As volume one covers 12 months of journey, volume 2 covers 6 months. Well, volume 3 covers 4 months. The speed is building up and increasing, steadily. This is volume 4, RISING, after breaking the sound barrier. Dr. Bak has reached a state where he is above most resistance and friction, he is now in a universe of his own, discovering his powers as he walks his journeys. This is no fiction story or wishful thinking, THE POWER OF YES is the journey of Dr. Bak, from one world record to the next, from one book to the next. You too can walk your own legend, you just need to listen to your innersole and open up to the opportunity. May you get inspiration from the legendary journey of Dr. Bak and find your own Destiny. Welcome to the Alphas.

THE RISE OF THE UNICORN -038
BY Dr. BAK NGUYEN & Dr. JEAN DE SERRES

In THE RISE OF THE UNICORN, Dr. Bak is joining forces with his friend and mentor, Dr. Jean De Serres. Together both men had many achievements in their respective industries, but the advent of eHappyPedia, THE RISE OF THE UNICORN is a personal project dear to both of them: the QUEST OF HAPPINESS and its empowerment. This book is a special one since you are witnessing the conversation between two entrepreneurs looking to change the world by building unique tools and media. Just like any enterprise, the ride is never a smooth one in the park on a beautiful day. But this is about eHappyPedia, it is about happiness, right? So it will happen and with a smile attached to it! The unique value of this book is that you are sharing the ups and downs of the launch of a Unicorn, not just the glory of the fame, but also the doubts and challenges along the way. May it inspire you on your own journey to success and happiness.

THE RISE OF THE UNICORN 2 -076
eHappyPedia
BY Dr. BAK NGUYEN & Dr. JEAN DE SERRES

This is 2 years after starting the first tome. Dr. Bak's brand is picking up, between the accumulation of records and recognition. eHappyPedia is now hot for a comeback. In THE RISE OF THE UNICORN 2, Dr. Bak is retracing and addressing each of Dr. Jean De Serres' concerns about the weakness of the first version of eHappyPedia and the eHappy movement. This is the sort of creation and a UNICORN both in finance and in psychology. Never before, have you assisted in such a daily and decision-making process of a world phenomenon and of a company. Dr. Bak and Dr. De Serres are literally using the process of writing this series of books to plan and brainstorm the birth of a bluechip. More than an intriguing story, this is the journey of 2 experienced entrepreneurs changing the world.

THE U.A.X STORY -072
THE ULTIMATE AUDIO EXPERIENCE
BY Dr. BAK NGUYEN

This is the story of the ULTIMATE AUDIO EXPERIENCE, U.A.X. Follow Dr. Bak's footsteps in how he invented a new way to read and learn. Dr. Bak brings his experience as a movie producer and a director to elevate the reading experience to another level with entertaining value and make it accessible to everyone, auditive, and visual people alike.

After three years plus of research and development, and countless hours of trials and errors, Dr. Bak finally solved his puzzle: having written more than 1.1 million words. The irony is that he does not like to read, he likes audiobooks! U.A.X. finally allowed the opening of Dr. Bak's entire library to a new genre and media. U.A.X. is the new way to learn and enjoy Audiobooks. Made to be entertaining while keeping the self-educational value of a book, U.A.X. will appeal to both auditive and visual people. U.A.X. is the blockbuster of Audiobooks. The format has already been approved by iTunes, Amazon, Spotify, and all major platforms for global distribution and streaming.

THE VACCINE -077
BY Dr. BAK NGUYEN & WILLIAM BAK

In THE VACCINE, A TALE OF SPIES AND ALIENS, Dr. Bak reprises his role as mentor to William, his 10-year-old son, both as co-author and as doctor. William is living through the COVID war and has accumulated many, many questions. That morning, they got out all at once. From a conversation between father and son, Dr. Bak is making science into words keeping the interest of his son on a Saturday morning in bed. William is not just an audience, he is responsible to map the field with his questions. What started as a morning conversation between father and son, became within the next hour, a great project, their 23rd book together. Learn about the virus, and vaccination while entertaining your kids.

TIMING - TIME MANAGEMENT ON STEROIDS 074
BY Dr. BAK NGUYEN & WILLIAM BAK

In TIMING, TIME MANAGEMENT ON STEROIDS, Dr. Bak is sharing his secret to keep overachieving, and overdelivering while raising the bar higher and higher. We all have 24 hours in a day, so how can some do so much more than others? Dr. Bak is not only sharing his secrets and mindset about time and efficiency, he is literally living his own words as this book is written within his last sprint to set the next world record of writing 100 books within 4 years, with only 31 days to go. With 8 books to write in 31 days, that's a little less than 4 days per book! Share the journey of a man surfing the change and looking to see where is the limit of the human mind, writing. In the meantime, understand his leverage, mindset, and secrets to challenge your own limits and dreams.

TO OVERACHIEVE EVERYTHING BEING LAZY -090
CHEAT YOUR WAY TO SUCCESS
BY Dr. BAK NGUYEN

In TO OVERACHIEVE EVERYTHING BEING LAZY, Dr. Bak retakes his role talking to the millennials, the next generation. If in the first tome of the series LAZY, Dr. Bak addresses the general audience of millennials, especially young women, he is dedicating this tome to the ALPHA amongst the millennials, those aiming for the moon and looking, not only to be happy but to change the world. This is not another take on how to cheat your way to success or how to leverage laziness, but this is the recipe to build overachievers and rainmakers. For the young leaders with ambitions and talent, understanding TIME and ENERGY are crucial from your first steps in writing your our legend. If Dr. Bak had the chance to do it all over again, this is how he would do it! Welcome to the Alphas.

TORNADO -067
FORCE OF CHANGE
BY Dr. BAK NGUYEN

In TORNADO - FORCE OF CHANGE Dr. Bak is writing solo. In the midst of the COVID war, change is not a good intention anymore. Change, constant change has become a new reality, a new norm. From somebody who holds the title of Industries' Disruptor, how does he yield change to stay in control? Well, the changes from the COVID war are constant fear and much loss of individual liberty. Some can endure the change, some will ride it. Dr. Bak is sharing his angle of navigating the changes, yielding the improvisations, and to reinvent the goals, the means to stay relevant. From fighting to keep his companies Dr. Bak went on to let go of the uncontrollable to embrace the opportunity, he reinvented himself to ride the change and create opportunities from an unprecedented crisis. This is the story of a man refusing to kneel and accept defeat, smiling back at faith to find leverage and hope.

TOUCHSTONE -073
LEVERAGING TODAY'S PSYCHOLOGICAL SMOG
BY Dr. BAK NGUYEN & Dr. KEN SEROTA

TOUCHSTONE, LEVERAGING TODAY'S PSYCHOLOGICAL SMOG is mapping to navigate and thrive in today's high and constant stress environment. After 40 years in practice, Dr. Serota is concerned about the evolution of the career of health care professionals and the never-ending level of stress. What is stress, and what are its effects, damages, and symptoms? If

COVID-19 revealed to the world that we are fragile, it also revealed most of the broken and the flaws of our system. For now a century, dentistry has been a champion in depression, Drug addiction, and suicide rates, and the curve is far from flattening. Dr. Bak is sharing his perspective and experience dealing with stress and how to leverage it into a constructive force. From the stress of a doctor with no right to failure to the stress of an entrepreneur never knowing the future, Dr. Bak is sharing his way to use stress as leverage.

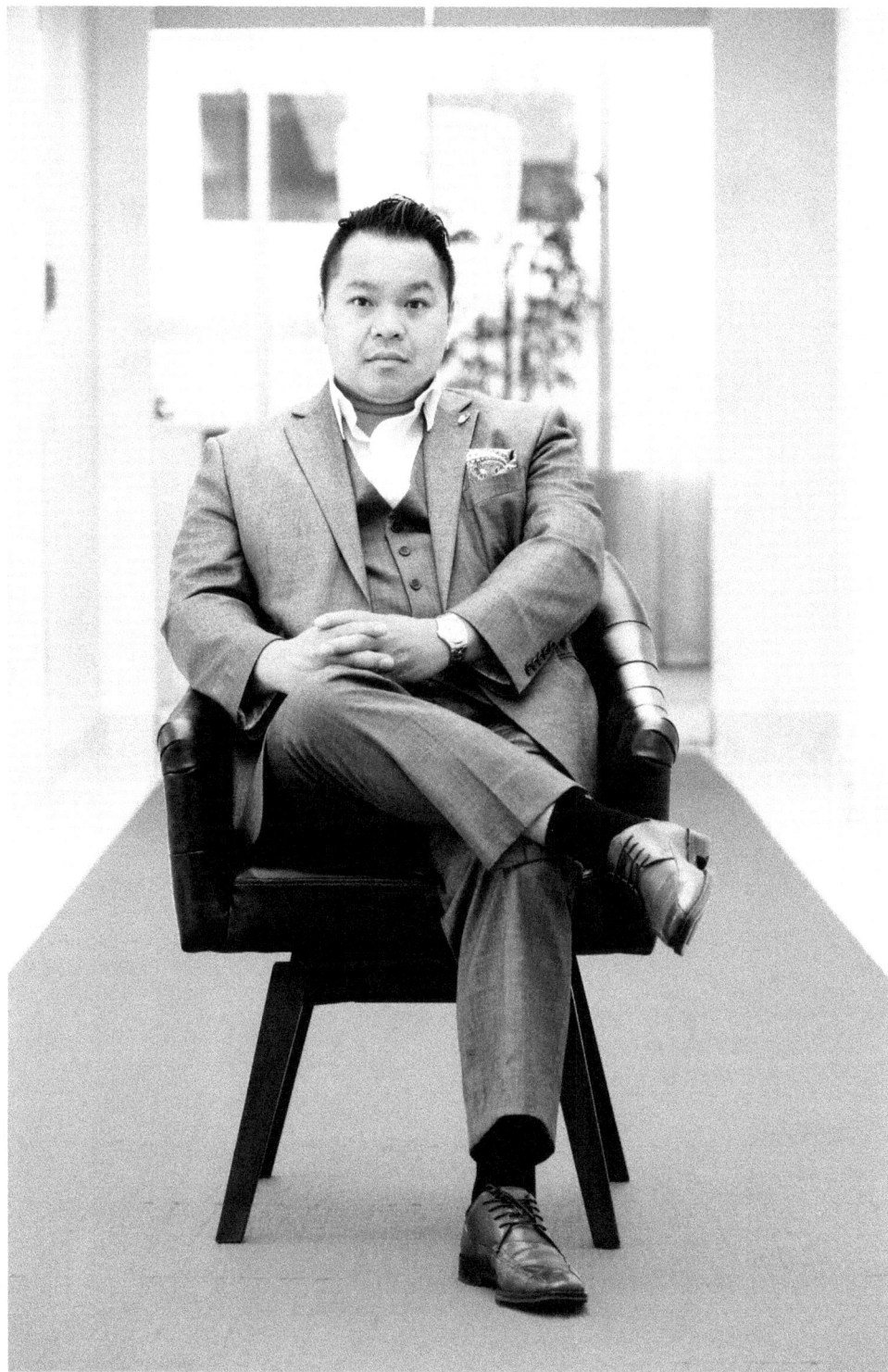

ABOUT THE CO-AUTHORS

From Canada, **Dr. BAK NGUYEN**, Nominee Ernst and Young Entrepreneur of the year, Grand Homage Lys DIVERSITY, LinkedIn & TownHall Achiever of the year and TOP 100 Doctors 2021. In 2023, he made the CREA GLOBAL AWARD list. Dr. Bak is a cosmetic dentist, CEO and founder of Mdex & Co. His company is revolutionizing the dental field.

Speaker and motivator, he holds the world record of writing 120 books in 5 years accumulating many world records (to be officialized). Before that, he held the world record of writing 9 books over 12 months, then, 15 books within 15 months to set the bar even higher with the world record of 36 books written within 18 months + 1 week.

By his second author anniversary, he scored his new landmark world record of 48 books within 24 months. And then 72 books in 36 months. By the 4th anniversary, Dr. Bak scored his usual landmark of writing 96 books over 48 months, but he pushed even further, scoring also the landmark world record of 100 books written within 4 years and then, 120 books written in 5 years! His books are covering:

ENTREPRENEURSHIP - LEADERSHIP - QUEST OF IDENTITY - DENTISTRY AND MEDICINE - PARENTING - CHILDREN BOOKS - PHILOSOPHY

In 2003, he founded Mdex, a dental company upon which in 2018, he launched the most ambitious private endeavour to reform the dental industry, Canada-wide. Philosopher, he has close to his heart the quest of happiness of the people surrounding him, patients and colleagues alike. In 2020, he launched an International collaborative initiative named **THE ALPHAS** to share knowledge and for Entrepreneurs and Doctors to thrive through the Greatest Pandemic and Economic depression of our time.

In 2016, he co-found with Tranie Vo, Emotive World Incorporated, a tech research company to use technology to empower happiness and sharing. U.A.X. the ultimate audio experience is the landmark project on which the team is advancing, utilizing the technics of the movie industry and the advancement in ARTIFICIAL INTELLIGENCE to save the book industry and upgrade the continuing education space.

These projects have allowed Dr. Nguyen to attract interest from the international and diplomatic community and he is now the centre of a global discussion on the wellbeing and the future of the health profession. It is in that matter that he shares his thoughts and encourages the health community to share their own stories. Motivational speaker and serial entrepreneur, philosopher and author, in his own words, Dr. Nguyen describes himself as a dentist by circumstances, an entrepreneur by nature and a communicator by passion. He also holds recognitions from the Canadian Parliament and the Canadian Senate.

From SPAIN, **Dr. MAHSA KHAGHANI**, Doctor of Dental Surgery, founder and CEO of BeIDE, a continuous educational platform for dentists. Experienced clinician in orthodontics, periodontal surgery and dental implant surgery, Dr. Khaghani is also leading a team of 30+ dentists in Madrid, Spain. Graduated from UCM (1999), member of the Illustrious College of Dentists of Madrid. Dr. Khaghani thrives on acquiring new knowledge and sharing them. She is the International Program Director at New York University and at PGO in Europe. She is a strong presence in the International Dental community and a leader for women and education. Ambassador in Spain of Digital dentistry society, clean implant foundation and SlowDentistry.

Degree in Dentistry from the UCM (1999), Member 28005521 of the Illustrious College of Dentists of Madrid, Invisalign Specialist, Specialist in Implantology and Periodontology. Diploma in Soft Tissue Management in Implantology taught by Dr. Sascha Jovanovic at the Branemark Center in Lleida (2011). Advanced continuing education in Implantology and Periodontology from New York University (NY 2009-2010). Diploma in advanced periodontics from the UCM (2010). Advanced treatments in periodontics and implantology. (2010), Advanced Course on Surgical Techniques and Aesthetic Implantology, Dr. Markus Hürzeler and Dr. Otto Zuhr. (2009), Esthetic surgery in Periodontal and implant dentistry, Dr. Markus Hürzeler and Dr. Otto Zuhr. (2009), Advanced Implantology course. Dr. Padrós. (2007), Implantology and Tissue Regeneration. Straumann. (2007), Oral Implant surgery course. European Dental Institute. (2006), Aesthetic Implantology and Oral Rehabilitation course. Dr. Julian Cuesta. (2006), Course on Porcelain Veneers and Aesthetic anterior groups. Dr. José A. from Rábago Vega. Ceosa. (2003-2004), Expert in Straight arch Orthodontics, Cervera (2001-2003), Dental Treatment in Special Patients. (2000), Numerous continuing training courses by different lecturers, nationally and internationally. Member of SEPES, SEPA, SE

From HUNGARY, **Dr. & Prof. KATALIN NAGY**, DDS; Ph.D; DSc. Head of Oral Surgery, Faculty of Dentistry University of Szeged, President of the Hungarian Dental Association, Secretary of the Hungarian Dental Professional Advisory Committee, Co-President of the Hungarian Implantology Association, Past president of the Hungarian Fulbright Association, Honorary Consul of Colombia. Professor Nagy did her specialty-degrees (in Oral Surgery, Prosthodontics, and Implantology) at the University of Szeged. She defended her Ph.D. and habilitation at the same place. She was appointed as the first Dean of The Dental Faculty, then she became the Vice President of the University of Szeged. Her main field of research is oral cancer. She defended her theses and received the title of DSc., at the Hungarian Academy of Science.

She speaks fluent English and German and basic Spanish. She gained her international academic experiences in different international Institutions, where she has spent a longer period of time (UK, United States, Germany, Finland). She is organizing the most prestigious Dental Conferences in the last

15 years in Hungary, and also she was the President of the ADEE. Professor Nagy is currently a full Professor and the Head of Oral Surgery at the University of Szeged, the President of the Hungarian Dental Association. She is the Honorary Consul of Colombia in Hungary.

ABOUT THE GUEST-AUTHORS

From the USA, **Dr. & Prof. PAUL DOMINIQUE** is a paediatric dentist, entrepreneur and investor. He's a graduate of the National University of Ireland, where he earned a Bachelor of Science degree in cell biology and molecular genetics. He completed his dental degree at the University of Kentucky and his specialty training in paediatrics at the Eastman Institute for Oral Health, University of Rochester, NY. Dr. Dominique served as an assistant professor in public health at the University of Kentucky, division of oral health science. During his tenure, he headed and improved a novel mobile program that successfully addresses access to care issues for children in Central and Western Kentucky.

Dr. Dominique is also an entrepreneur having acquired and consolidated a small group of practices growing from less than 700K to over 2.4 Million EBITDA in under 24 months. Dr. Dominique has been angel investing for the past decade, investing across a diverse group of platforms such as equity crowdfunding, psychedelic medicine, real estate and teledentistry. He currently serves as a board advisory member to the Teledentists and Revere Partners, the first venture fund dedicated to oral health. He's currently involved in a project that is exploring the use of blockchain technology and NFTs to help improve access to dental care. Dr. Dominique joined the Alphas in 2020 as he contributed to the Teledentistry Summit at the beginning of the COVID crisis. Since Dr. Dominique has contributed to many Alphas summits and books including RELEVANCY and the ALPHA DENTISTRY book franchise (volumes 1 and 4).

From the USA, **Dr. & Prof. PAUL OUELLETTE**, DDS, MS, ABO, AFAAID, WORLD TOP 100 DOCTOR 2020, Former Associate Professor Georgia School of Orthodontics and Jacksonville University. Highly motivated to help my sons become successful in the "Ouellette Family of Dentists" Group Dental Specialty Practice. During the Pandemic, Dr. Ouellette was amongst the co-founders of the ALPHAS. He also advances his research in the field of mobile dentistry and makes the practice of dentistry affordable and accessible to everyone from everywhere. Dr. Ouellette has contributed to many Alphas summits and books including RELEVANCY, MIDAS TOUCH, THE POWER OF DR, AMONGST THE ALPHAS, KISS ORTHODONTICS and the ALPHA DENTISTRY book franchise.

From the USA, **Dr. ARASH HAKHAMIAN**, DDS, is a Doctor of Dental Surgery based in Los Angeles, California. He has been practicing dentistry since 2010 and is a graduate of the University of Southern California with a degree in

Doctor of Dental Surgery. Dr. Arash is recognized and respected in his field and is known for teaching dentists advanced clinical procedures, as well as providing life-changing dentistry to his patients locally and internationally. With over a decade of experience in the field, he is the founder and CEO of Dentulu, the world's leading tele-dentistry company which was awarded the Best Tele-dentistry Technology two times at the American Dental Association. As the CEO of Dentulu, Dr. Hakhamian has helped to revolutionize the field of tele-dentistry, developing innovative technologies and services that enable dental professionals to provide care remotely. Dentulu's platform provides patients with access to a wide range of dental services, including virtual consultations, at-home dental exams, and remote monitoring. Dr. Hakhamian is committed to continuing to innovate and drive the field of tele-dentistry forward, ensuring that patients around the world have access to high-quality dental care, regardless of their location or financial resources. In addition to his practice, he was a co-founder of the Global Dental Implant Academy and serves on the board of directors at the International Extraction Academy.

From the USA, **Dr. MARILYN SANDOR**, DDS, MS, is one of Southwest Florida's favourite paediatric dentists. She is highly experienced in her field, having founded her private practice, Naples Paediatric Dentistry in the beautiful community of Naples, Florida in 2001. Dr. Sandor is a successful business owner and an active member of her community. She is committed to educating her young patients on the importance of oral health and enjoys teaching children how to have healthy smiles for a lifetime. Dr. Sandor's paediatric-focused invention, Zooby prophy angles, inspired a full line of creative new products by Young Innovations which have been bringing joy to dental patients around the world for over a decade. She is the founder and CEO of GOODCHECKUP is the first Mobile to Mobile, Patent pending, Teledentistry solution that, gives dentists everywhere the ability to set themselves free from the standard care model and provide patients total convenience by placing access to care at their fingertips.

From Albania, **Dr. & Prof. GURIEN DEMIRAQI**, DDS, MS, PhD, FIADFE is a dental professional who specializes in oral surgery, OMF surgery, oral anesthetics, and implantology. Graduated in dentistry in the Faculty of Dentistry, Tirana University in 2003. From 2003-2006 specialized in Oral surgery and Implantology with DDS, BwKh Berlin (University hospital of Charite) and OMF Surgery, BwKh Amberg (University hospital of Friedrich-Alexander- Universität Erlangen-Nürnberg) Germany, BwzKh Koblenz (University hospital of Johannes Gutenberg University-Mainz) Germany. From 2007, pedagogue and lecturer in oral surgery; OMF surgery; oral anesthetics and implantology in the Dentistry Department, Faculty of Medical Sciences of the Albanian University.

From 2009-2015 chef of OMF surgery cathedra in the Dentistry Department, Faculty of Medical Sciences of the Albanian University. From 2010 Master and later PHD in oral implantology in the Faculty of Dentistry, Tirana University with the theme "Oral and systemic pathologies that affect the osteointegration of implants, a comparative study of several implant systems used in Albania". Speaker in and outside Albania in important events. Author and coauthor of many articles in Albanian and international magazines concerning oral and maxillofacial surgery, orthodontics, endodontics and implantology. Board editor of several scientific magazines. Organizer of courses in grafting, implantology at different levels, accelerated orthodontics and endodontics. Maintains the private practice at the clinic "DemiraqiDental" in Tirana, Albania. General director of the OMF diagnostic center Grafi Dentare Skanner 3D Galeria. Inventor of the "Sticky Tooth" grafting material, Co-inventor of the Baruti-Demiraqi approach, a PAOO enhancement technique with hard and soft tissue grafting protocol. Member of European Association for Osteointegration (EAO), World Dental Federation (FDI), South Europe North Africa Middle East Society of Implantology and Modern Dentistry (SENAME), Balkan Stomatological Society (BASS), Member and Expert of the International Extraction Academy (IEA) and Global Implantology Institute (GII), Awarded Top 100 Doctor in Dentistry in 2020 by the Global Summits Institute (GSI) and later Chair of the Scientific Committee of GSI, currently Regent of the Global Summits Institute (GSI), member of the International Ambassador Committee of the Academy of Oral Surgery (AOS), Member and Albanian President of the International Academy of Implantoprosthesis and Osteoconnection (IAIO), Fellow of the International Academy for Dental-Facial Esthetics (IADFE), Visiting professor at the Universal School of Health in the University of California, Opinion Leader of several dentistry firms etc. Major areas of interest include oral and maxillofacial surgery, implantology, accelerated orthodontics, guided regeneration, endodontic surgery, growth factors, emergency profiles in implantology and so on.

From MALAYSIA, **Dr. & Prof. BENNETE FERNANDES**, BDS, MDS, PhD (h.c.), is a periodontist with 18 years of academic and clinical experience. He completed his graduation (BDS) from KVG Dental College and Hospital, Sullia, Karnataka and obtained a Master degree in Periodontology from JSS Dental College and Hospital, Mysuru, under the agies of the prestigious Rajiv Gandhi University of Health Sciences (RGUHS), Bengaluru, India in 2004. He has done his Fellowship in Implantology from Nobel Biocare and also his Fellowship in LASER dentistry from Genoa University, Italy. He was awarded an honorary PhD. degree in 2021 by the International Internship University (IIU) and another honorary PhD. degree in 2022 by Wisdom University, Nigeria. He is a Fellow of Pierre Fauchard Academy (FPFA) ; Fellow of International College of Continuing Dental Education (FICCDE), Fellow of Academia Internacional De Odontologia Integral (FAIOI), Fellow of The Royal Society of Public Health (FRSPH) from UK, Fellow of The Royal Society of Medicine (RSM)- Odontology Section from UK, Fellow of The Royal Academy of Medicine (RAMI)- Odontology Section from Ireland. He had worked for around 11 years in India before moving to the Faculty of Dentistry, SEGi University, Malaysia since the last 7 years.

From BRAZIL, **Dr. & Prof. SANDRA FABIANO**, DDS, MSC, is a Periodontics and Oral Implantology specialist in private practice in Rio de Janeiro, Brazil. She graduated in Dentistry from Valença Dental School in Rio de Janeiro and completed her specialization in Periodontics at the Brazilian Dental

Association (ABO) in Rio de Janeiro. She also completed a continuous education course in Periodontics at the University of Texas Dental Branch in Houston. Her training in Implant Dentistry was provided by Nobel Biocare Brazil at Sendick Clinic in São Paulo. She earned her Master's degree (MSc) in Implantology from São Leopoldo Mandic Faculty in Campinas, São Paulo, Brazil, where she later served as an Assistant Professor in the Master Course in Oral Implantology. Dr. Sandra is currently the Coordinator Professor of specialization in Implant Dentistry at São Leopoldo Mandic Faculty, Campus Rio de Janeiro. She is an active member of the Brazilian Academy of Dentistry and her field of interest is guided bone regeneration, bone substitutes, autologous blood concentrates, and periodontal and peri-implant plastic surgeries. Dr. Sandra is also an active National and International speaker. She loves working at the University and considers it her mission to educate and inspire young female students at the beginning of their careers.

UAX

ULTIMATE AUDIO EXPERIENCE

A new way to learn and enjoy Audiobooks. Made to be entertaining while keeping the self-educational value of a book, UAX will appeal to both auditive and visual people. UAX is the blockbuster of Audiobooks.

UAX will cover most of Dr. Bak's books and is now negotiating to bring more authors and more titles to the UAX concept. Now streaming on Spotify, Apple Music and Amazon Prime. Available for download on all major music platforms. Give it a try today!

AMAZON · BARNES & NOBLE · APPLE BOOKS · KINDLE
SPOTIFY · APPLE MUSIC

C O M B O
PAPERBACK/AUDIOBOOK
ACTIVATION

Please register your book to receive the link to your audiobook version.
Register at:
https://baknguyen.com/leadership-changing-the-world-registry

ALPHA DENTISTRY vol. 3 -132
PAEDIATRIC DENTISTRY FAQ
INTERNATIONAL EDITION

ENGLISH ARABIC FRANÇAIS ITALIAN SPANISH
BY Dr. BAK NGUYEN, Dr. PAUL DOMINIQUE, Dr.
RICHARD SIMPSON, Dr. AURORA ALVA, Dr. NOUR
AMMAR, Dr. AILIN CABRERA-MATTA, Dr. NIDHI TANEJA,
Dr. PIERLUIGI PELAGALLI, Dr. PRRIYA PORWAL

ALPHA DENTISTRY vol. 4 -135
PAEDIATRIC DENTISTRY FAQ
ASSEMBLED EDITION

ALBANIA AUSTRALIA CANADA GERMANY INDIA
IRAN MALAYSIA SPAIN USA
BY Dr. BAK NGUYEN, Dr. ERIC LACOSTE, Dr. MAZIAR
SHAHZAD DOWLATSHAHI, Dr. BENNETE FERNANDES,
Dr. MEENU BHASIN, Dr. HASTEE BHANUSHALI, Dr.
ROBERT M. PICK, Dr. AMIN MOTAMEDI, Dr. TIHANA
DIVNIC-RESNIK, Dr. ARNE VON STERNHEIM, Dr.
FERNANDO ARPÓN MORENO and Dr. GURIEN
DEMIRAQI

ALPHA DENTISTRY vol. 4 -136
PAEDIATRIC DENTISTRY FAQ
INTERNATIONAL EDITION

ENGLISH FRENCH GERMAN HINDI ITALIAN
MANDARIN MALAY ARABIC SPANISH SHQIP
BY Dr. BAK NGUYEN, Dr. ERIC LACOSTE, Dr. MAZIAR
SHAHZAD DOWLATSHAHI, Dr. BENNETE FERNANDES,
Dr. MEENU BHASIN, Dr. HASTEE BHANUSHALI, Dr.
ROBERT M. PICK, Dr. AMIN MOTAMEDI, Dr. TIHANA
DIVNIC-RESNIK, Dr. ARNE VON STERNHEIM, Dr.
FERNANDO ARPÓN MORENO and Dr. GURIEN
DEMIRAQI

ALPHA DENTISTRY vol. 5 -137
PAEDIATRIC DENTISTRY FAQ
ASSEMBLED EDITION

AUSTRALIA CANADA FRANCE LITHUANIA PERU
TURKEY UKRAINE USA
BY Dr. BAK NGUYEN, Dr. JULIO REYNAFARJE, Dr. LINA
DUSEVIČIŪTĖ, Dr. NAZARIY MYKHAYLYUK, Dr. CLAUDE

MOUAFO, Dr. MANOJ RAJAN, Dr. LOUIS KAUFMAN, Dr.
LILIAN SHI and Dr. YASEMIN OZKAN

ALPHA DENTISTRY vol. 5 -138
PAEDIATRIC DENTISTRY FAQ
INTERNATIONAL EDITION

ENGLISH ARABIC FRENCH LITHUANIAN
SPANISH UKRAINIAN
BY Dr. BAK NGUYEN, Dr. JULIO REYNAFARJE, Dr. LINA
DUSEVIČIŪTĖ, Dr. NAZARIY MYKHAYLYUK, Dr. CLAUDE
MOUAFO, Dr. MANOJ RAJAN, Dr. LOUIS KAUFMAN, Dr.
LILIAN SHI and Dr. YASEMIN OZKAN

QUEST OF IDENTITY

IDENTITY -004
THE ANTHOLOGY OF QUESTS
BY Dr. BAK NGUYEN

HYBRID -011
THE MODERN QUEST OF IDENTITY
BY Dr. BAK NGUYEN

PARENTING

THE ORIGIN SERIES

with William Bak

LEGENDS OF DESTINY

THE POWER OF YES

UNLIMITED ACCESS
DR. BAK'S ENTIRE AUDIO LIBRARY

Since Dr. Bak set his new landmark world record of writing 100 books in 4 years, he is opening his entire audio library, audiobooks and UAX albums, exclusively to all VIP members for $9.99/month.

By becoming a VIP member, you will have access to all Dr. Bak's audiobooks and UAX albums. Those are the ones today bought at Apple Books, Audible, and in COMBO version at Amazon. The UAX albums are those streaming on Apple Music, Spotify, and Amazon Prime Music.

As a VIP, you will also have prime access to the audiobooks as soon as they are completed, hitting them before they reach the mainstream outlets. Get your membership today!

http://drbaknguyen.com/members

Welcome to the Alphas.

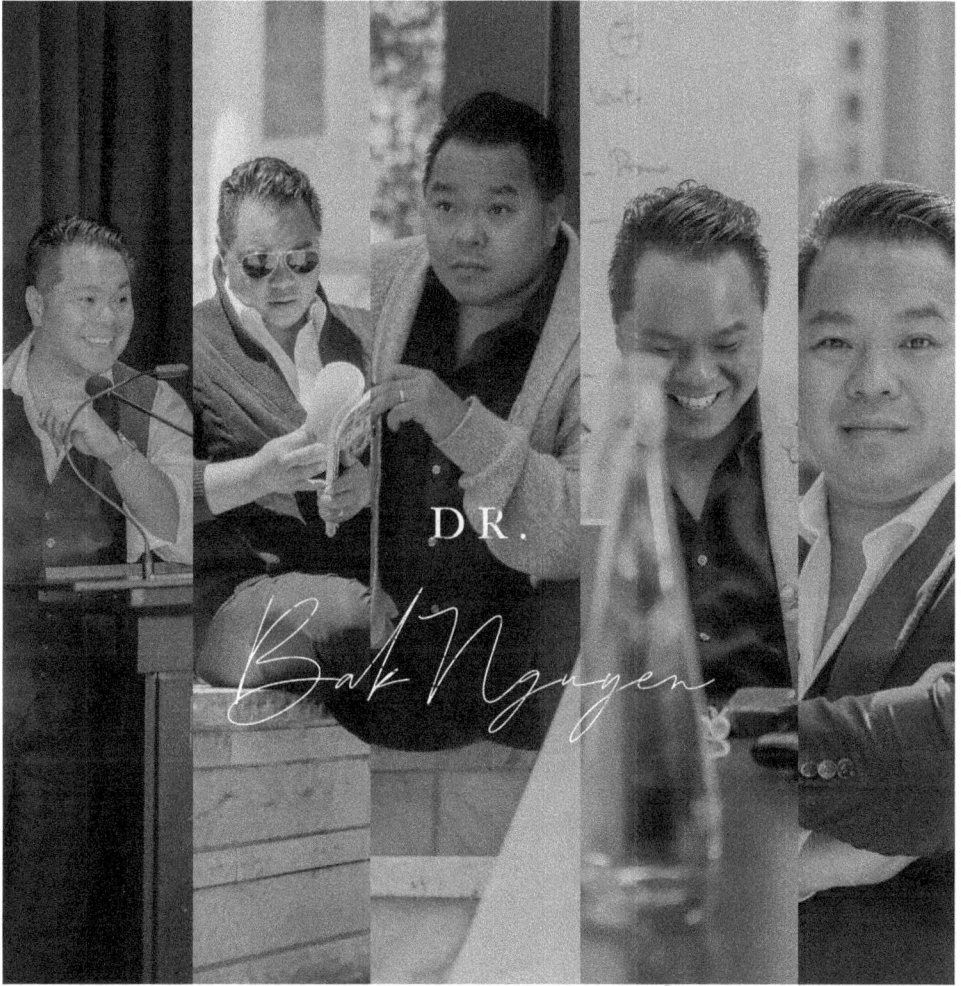

DR.

Bak Nguyen